FEARFULLY
AND
WONDERFULLY
MADE:

The HEART of the Matter!

Why Heart Attacks Happen And
A Plan For Living Well After The Event

FEARFULLY AND WONDERFULLY MADE:

The HEART of the Matter!

Why Heart Attacks Happen And
A Plan For Living Well After The Event

DR. CAROL S. IGHOFOSE

WOW Book Publishing™

Dedication

"In loving memory of my dear Mother, Edna Douglas (nee McKenzie). You never lived to witness my accomplishments beyond my 10th birthday, but your health career aspirations became mine."

Testimonials

"Thoughtful, perceptive and inspirational. Carol has proved herself masterfully adept at turning a potentially tragic situation into a positive and enlightening narrative that will move the heart of every reader. A classic tale of triumph in the face of adversity—amazing!"

—Dr. T. L. Bempah

"I applaud Carol's endeavour to tackle this expansive but highly interesting subject matter: The Heart. By writing the book: "Fearfully and Wonderfully Made", Carol has taken her own negative experience and turned it into a positive. This book opens up new and compelling chapters that are intriguing and informative. I am sure they will make an impact on many lives. Hats off to her!"

—Reverend D. S. Hunter

"When I started reading the book, I couldn't put it down. I wanted to know what happened next. I found the medical explanations fascinating as I had never given "my heart" much thought. I now have a good understanding of its construction and how it "works". Also, what an Amazing and Awesome God we have! The quotes from The Holy Bible were much appreciated. Thank you for this very helpful book Dr. Carol. I look forward to the next one!"

—Norma V. Moore

"Dr Carol Ighofose's book is literally a heartfelt response to the myocardial infarction—the heart attack—that she suffered out of the blue in 2018. She interweaves medical information with her own personal testimony throughout a text that is part narrative, part medical explanation and above all a manifestation of her burning desire to offer Christian comfort to fellow heart attack survivors. She shows how many vital factors, including her own personal faith, have helped and strengthened the healing process, and I am convinced that her story will be a source of solace to others who have undergone similarly unexpected trauma. Dr Ighofose offers practical and spiritual advice to those who are recovering from heart-related illnesses in a book which will enable men and women who have had an unforeseen brush with darkness to live again."

—Simon Mold

Contents

Acknowledgements xi

Why You Should Read this Book xiii

Introduction 1

Chapter 1: The Heart Of The Matter!.....................................5

Chapter 2: The Attack! 11

Chapter 3: Accident And Emergency Department................. 21

Chapter 4: Glenfield Hospital/Coronary Care Unit............... 31

Chapter 5: Risk Factors For Myocardial Infarction 37

Chapter 6: Complications Of Myocardial Infarction............. 45

Chapter 7: Structure And Function Of The Heart 49

Chapter 8: Management After A Myocardial Infarction........ 61

Chapter 9: The Psychological And Spiritual Impact Of
Myocardial Infarction 67

Chapter 10: Moving Forward After A Myocardial
Infarction—Practical Issues 83

Chapter 11: Fearfully And Wonderfully Made........................ 93

Glossary Of Terms... 102

About The Author 105

Acknowledgements

I acknowledge Jesus Christ, the one I believe to be God in the flesh, who now dwells in me in the form of the Holy Spirit, providing me with ongoing guidance, comfort, and empowerment.

My mother Edna is no longer with us, but she would be extremely proud of this work. My father Hartlan planted the seed of hard work in my psyche through his example and countless labours of love for his children.

My husband Simon for his ongoing love and support and my two princes Emmanuel and Caleb who always elicit visceral guffaws from me or bring a gentle smile to my face and tell me I am the best mother ever!

My amazing siblings, Debbie, Andrea and Winston. Words can't express my love for you guys. We've been on a long journey together! By extension, my wonderful nieces and nephews have made the ride that much more enjoyable!

My pastor and his wife, Elder D. S. and Evangelist D. Hunter as well as all the members of Bethel Pneuma Tabernacle Church (Apostolic) in Leicester, UK. The regional, national and international Bethel Apostolic Church family have also provided me with countless and ongoing prayers and support, for which I am eternally grateful.

My angels: amazing friend and adopted sister-Trace (Dr. Tracey Bempah); adopted mother, sister, friend and 'Fairy Godmother'—Sister Ivy (Mrs. Herma Hamilton); my doting adopted big sister—Jenny (Miss Jennifer Solomon); my marvellous and attentive in-laws—Mum (Norma), Mehdi, Margaret, Ian, Jacqui and Aunty Margo. You are all absolute treasures!

My wonderful GP colleagues and friends who supported me in the most awesome and pragmatic ways, you are true healers! My other amazing work colleagues—you know who you are, your support and cheeky messages have also helped me heal!

Thanks also to all the Health Care staff members who were involved in my care and contributed in some way to ensuring that I am still here to write this book.

Special thanks to the British Heart Foundation (BHF) for permitting me to include material from their website in this book.

Why you should read this book

This book will provide you with:

- A reminder of the physical and spiritual make up of our amazing human body and the love and desire of God our creator, to heal and restore us—even if it takes a miracle!

- An overview of the heart's structure and function and what happens during and after a heart attack.

- Advice from a practising Christian GP on how to take care of our physical body as well as our psychological and spiritual wellbeing.

- A perspective that will provoke thoughtfulness regarding the debate on creation and evolution.

Introduction

If you are reading this, you have either survived or know someone who has had a heart attack. If you are a survivor—well done! Thank God you are still here and welcome to the club!

As a medically trained member of the survivors' club, I realise that my insight may prove useful to helping you understand why this has happened to you or your loved one and help you see that living well after a heart attack is indeed possible! Don't worry; your life is not over yet! However, you will need to learn a few things to help you live well, now that you have 'a heart condition'.

I also want to share my account of surviving what in medical terms is known as a myocardial infarction (MI) or heart attack in common speak. By doing so, I hope to open up the language that we doctors use to provide you the vocabulary to discuss your condition with your GP and/or consultant, or any other healthcare professional you may wish to interact with in an informed way.

By the way, the ability to confidently articulate knowledge about your condition along with symptoms and treatment concerns you have, may improve your chance of receiving a better quality of care. This is because healthcare professionals recognise the "Expert Patient"- trust me, I'm a doctor!

My heart attack stopped me in my tracks! I am a busy GP, wife, mother, sister, and aunty—family "matriarch" (having taken on the mother's role to my 3 siblings after losing our mother when I was only 10 years old). I am also a Sunday School Teacher, Women's Ministry Leader, Charity Trustee and Church Secretary. As a trusted confidante, I am an 'agony aunt' to many of my friends, whom I love dearly and appreciate for their reciprocal encouragement and support.

I was working on average a 50-hour week, which often included a Saturday night 8pm to 8am shift. I would then get up for church after only 2 hours sleep and present the Sunday School lesson from 1pm for at least an hour if not more. I also often volunteer my time to give presentations on various health topics to community and church groups of various sizes. Despite my busy work schedule, I am always cognizant of maintaining a good 'work-life balance' and would usually reserve Mondays as my rest and relaxation days. Two months prior to my heart attack, I realised that I was doing too much and felt that it might adversely impact my health and so dropped the Saturday night shifts, to the delight of my husband! Does this sound familiar?

Winding up in the Coronary Care Unit at the renowned Glenfield Hospital (GH) a specialist cardiac and respiratory care centre, I realised that my hectic lifestyle had finally come to a forceful stop when my Pastor, at my bedside, quoted a portion of verse 2 from Psalm 23—"He maketh me to lie down"!

This led me to pause and reflect once again on what I learnt during medical school—HOW AMAZING OUR HUMAN BODY IS and our responsibility to take care of it!

In this book, I will take you on a journey—examining the structure and function of the heart and its relationship to all other body structures, whilst describing my experience of this wonderful organ being 'broken' but surviving the trauma without ceasing to do what it does best—pump for life!

Though my heart suffered a temporary insult from being deprived of blood to certain parts, I envision its miraculous recovery. I compare the natural heart to the human soul, highlighting our threefold status as living beings possessing a body, soul and spirit. Hence, my definition of and the need to acknowledge and maintain holistic health, recognising that a heart attack not only affects our physical body, but also has psychological and spiritual implications.

In this book I will not shy away from looking at the practicalities of life after an MI, the possible complications and difficulties that I and my family could face in the future.

This book is the first in a series called 'Fearfully and Wonderfully Made' which will detail how the various body systems provide evidence for the amazing works of God, our creator. In essence, the planned series of books will provide a Christian medical perspective of the human body, whilst examining a system-related disease (known by medics as a pathology).

The major body systems to be explored in future books will include:

- The Central Nervous System (CNS)
- Ophthalmology (Eye)
- Ear, Nose and Throat (ENT)
- Respiratory
- Gastrointestinal
- Obstetrics and Gynaecology
- Musculoskeletal
- Genito-urinary
- Endocrine and immune system
- Integumentary/Dermatology (Skin)

CHAPTER 1

The Heart Of The Matter!

As we clear away boxes in our cold, gloomy attic following an impending house move, my thoughts are drawn back to my days at medical school at the University of Leicester. The folders containing countless notes on histology, genetics, cardiovascular system and biological molecules are making themselves seen as they are moved from their long-forgotten resting place. For years, they have been neatly packed in a box, thanks to my husband, and are now coated in spiders' webs and attic dust! I look at them with mixed feelings, reminiscing trepidation but also breathing a deep sigh of relief . . . *"Phew!! Thank God those days are behind me, but what an amazing 'machine' our human body is!"*

The lingering feeling of unfulfillment begins to rear its ugly head—*"I promised I would use those! Use them to write about the amazing human body and demonstrate how God formed us perfectly . . . The overarching title would be 'Fearfully and Wonderfully Made'"*. I have Miss Neeta to thank for this title. I recall her as a light-skinned, curly-haired Jamaican lady and my no-nonsense RE teacher, from sunnier, happy days spent at Edwin Allen Comprehensive High School in Jamaica, fondly called "Compre". She made me, and my classmates learn Psalm 139 by rote! Now I'm glad I did! *"Maybe I should"* I told myself. *"I will start the series soon— just need to complete these two books which I am currently working on!"* One of which was started over 9-years ago!

A few weeks pass after the house move and now my whole attention is focussed on my heart—that precious organ that started beating by the time the cells forming me in my mother Edna's womb were only 3 weeks old. It could be recognised as a heart a mere 8 weeks after my conception! *"Oh, the longevity of my heart! What an organ! 49 years later and it has never stopped! It has kept pumping all this time without fail . . . but it almost stopped 3 weeks ago! Suddenly! Out of the blue! And no one saw it coming! I certainly didn't!"*

"Now I know I have to start writing the series—starting with the cardiovascular system (CVS), of course . . . it's a 'no-brainer'! Never mind the other two books I've been working on—they can wait for now".

As far as I'm aware, my heart was in great condition. I have none of the usual risk factors for cardiovascular disease! I started enumerating a list in my head:

1. *No known personal or family history of cardiac/ coronary heart disease (CHD);*
2. *I have never smoked;*
3. *I'm not a drinker;*
4. *I have never done drugs;*
5. *My body weight is decent—Body Mass Index (BMI)*

of 26; technically slightly overweight if one is to be guided by the National Institute for Health and Care Excellence's (NICE) BMI classification of 25-29.9 being overweight but certainly nothing to gasp about! (Find more information on my website at www. ferafullyandwonderfully.org).

6. *I do my exercises regularly, though that could always be improved! Come to think of it, I hadn't been on my exercise machine since the house move a few weeks previously. The Maxi-climber was still lurking somewhere in the garage—waiting for my husband to extract and position it in an appropriate space so I could resume my exercise pattern. Nonetheless, I had been busy carrying things to and from the car, up and down stairs and my heart did have to do some serious work when I took a series of swimming lessons recently—"dear God, that swimming was some intense exercise!" However, upon reflection, the 8-mile round trip I would do daily as a child growing up in Jamaica to get to and from school was, by comparison, no contest to those swimming lessons!*

In Jamaica, the daily walking I did growing up was out of necessity; it certainly wasn't a lifestyle choice for health and fitness reasons! In those days walking was the only and NECESSARY means to my destination. As I got older, accessing the luxury of motorised transport to carry me to high school, involved an 8-mile trek, through country tracks to the nearest main road! The point is, my heart is accustomed to rigorous and prolonged hard work and I have never been one to have a sedentary lifestyle!

My list continued . . .

7. *No history of diabetes or high blood pressure (though I know I am at risk for both);*

8. *Cholesterol level normal below 5 mmol/l.*

This was a total shock! I anticipated that my heart would remain in great condition until well into my 80's at least! . . . *I had no need for regular medications and was going to keep it that way!* I have always envisioned myself remaining in fabulously good health into old age! I intended to enjoy every aspect of my life. I always had and still have a wariness about Type 2 Diabetes Mellitus (T2DM) and hypertension (high blood pressure) so consciously adopted a lifestyle to ward off both, simply because I have two risk factors, namely: family history and ethnicity. My maternal Grandma and my 1st cousin were both diagnosed with T2DM and my father has hypertension. Being a black Caribbean also puts me at increased risk for both conditions. In addition, age is now also a factor given that I am now over 40!

Anyway, I dream of taking all my future beautiful grandchildren (I laugh to myself as I think hopefully 6 of them!) to Jamaica—always travelling in First Class on the flights and ensuring my darlings enjoy the most amazing holidays. My dream was even more pleasurable as I relished the thought of being able to return them to their parents (my current teenage children!) once the holidays were over! But then, SUDDENLY, THE DREAM WAS DISRUPTED . . .

On 22nd January 2018, things changed dramatically and significantly! I suffered a Heart Attack- just under three weeks before my 49th birthday! My perfect heart . . . *"How did this happen? When did things go so wrong? Why is this happening to me?"*

I felt a slight discomfort in my epigastrium (stomach/upper abdomen) as I was about to leave work at around 12:45 pm—I recall the time clearly as I was running a bit late. I should have left 15 minutes earlier but was tying up events from my last telephone call and a quick chit chat to my colleague taking over the shift for the afternoon. *"Oh, a bit of indigestion,"* I thought, *"I'm fasting today -not eaten anything . . . will break my fast before my next shift starts at 4pm later today."* I got into my car and started the journey home.

A quick call to Si (my husband—Simon) using the car's Bluetooth system to let him know I'm on the way home. *"Oh, Tracey has been waiting to speak to me . . . she is still up after her night shift . . . must be dying to sleep. My darling friend, she is now living the junior doctor's life I left behind, and on the wards too, with those super hectic on-call night shifts; invariably short staffed—I remember those days . . . or nights!"* *"Strange though that she hasn't decided to go to bed and speak to me later after she has had some rest. Hmmm . . . I wonder why she has chosen to wait up all this time for me . . . ?"*

CHAPTER 2

The Attack!

I was still talking to Tracey via my car's Bluetooth hands free system, when I realised that my very mild 'indigestion' symptom was now a 'discomfort' of sort in the centre of my chest. "Trace," I said, "I've never had chest pain, but I have this discomfort in my chest . . . just telling you in case anything happens."

She was alarmed and went into 'doctor's mode': "Tell me more about the discomfort Carol. How exactly would you describe it? How much would you grade it on a scale of 1-10? . . . and so on . . ."

We chatted and agreed that I should get it checked out at some point—sooner rather than later. I made a mental note that I was not too far from the local A&E department. *"If this continues I'll just drive to A&E, park my car and go inside,"* I thought. Then Tracey hinted that she was about to change the subject and start discussing another matter.

I suddenly realised that I was not able to concentrate! "Trace," I said, "This is not right, I need to pull over." Tracey's now clearly panicked voice replied "Oh my God Carol, pull over, I'll call the ambulance! Where are you? What's your car licence number?" I was losing focus! "Never mind that!" I partially hissed, as I realised that it required far too much concentration to tell her my car registration number (of course I knew my number plate!). "Just tell them It's a BMW X5, it's a big car, they won't miss it! I am turning into Raw Dykes Road," I said, I was trying to tell her that I could see Leicester City Football club but couldn't find the right words to express this. In fact, I am not sure what I said as I pulled over and mounted the pavement to park the car out of harm's way and the oncoming traffic.

By this time the 'discomfort' had become a pain in the centre of my chest. I started sweating and felt clammy and dizzy. *"I need some fresh air,"* I thought, but somehow, I could not now work out how to lower my car windows.

Once the blood supply to the cardiac muscles becomes depleted, the resulting insult to that area of heart muscle means that the heart's pumping action is impaired, restricting the blood supply to other tissues and organs in the body including the brain. My disorientation or mild confused state meant that my brain was beginning to become starved of oxygen. I managed to work out which buttons to push to get my car windows lowered to bring fresh air into the car. I looked outside and saw people passing by, all of them completely oblivious to my predicament. I managed a wilted pathetic wave through the window in the hope that someone would stop and sit with me. It is at times like these that one realises the value of human company. The thought crossed my mind that it would be sad to die alone but that suggestion was promptly rebuked! I felt very reassured that I would not die despite being fully aware that this was a real possibility, especially as I was now convinced that I was having a heart attack!

My phone rang—it was still coming over the car Bluetooth system—It was Si. His voice was controlled but with the inevitable hint of anxiety *"Poor thing! I'm sure that he's more worried than he's making out."* Simon's voice hailed me over the car speaker, "Carol, are you ok? I'm on my way! Tracey called me. Don't panic. Cough as hard as you can!" he said, "keep coughing and don't stop until I get there!" I started coughing—recalling a WhatsApp chain-message we had both received, advising how coughing can mimic chest compressions (even if mildly) and may improve the cardiac blood flow in a heart attack. I still don't know if this is true! However, at the time, evidence-based practice was not my priority! I just kept coughing and talking to the Lord Jesus, thanking Him for being with me. I thought fondly of my two boys—my two princes! Oh, how I love those boys . . .

A heart attack describes an event which results in damage or death to the heart muscle because of no blood flow carrying nutrients and oxygen to that area of the heart. This is also referred to as a myocardial infarction (MI), as the affected heart muscle i.e. myocardium is infarcted—dies because of circulatory blood loss.

The lack of blood and oxygen to the heart muscles causes a sudden onset of pain or discomfort in the chest which persists. Sometimes the brain interprets this as indigestion or other non-specific pain especially if the individual involved had not previously experienced ischaemia (lack of blood supply) to the cardiac muscles; apparently, the brain is unsure how to interpret these new pain signals. This suggests that my heart attack might have actually started at the time when I was leaving work and thought that I was experiencing indigestion symptoms. Of course, at the time a heart attack was the furthest thing from my mind! Why on earth would I be thinking of that? I was perfectly fine!

During a heart attack, the pain may spread to the arms or up the neck and jaw—this is due to what we doctors call 'referred pain'. The nerves that supply the chest originate from an area that also supplies the arm, neck and jaw area. I later had referred pain to my left arm but again, it wasn't what I expected, initially—it felt rather like a numbing heaviness that was unexplained. Other associated signs and symptoms during a heart attack may include nausea (feeling 'sick') and/or vomiting, shortness of breath, excessive sweating, feeling faint and the individual may collapse. These signs and symptoms occur as a result of increased adrenaline from the 'fight or flight' response of the sympathetic nervous system activity of the Autonomic Nervous System (ANS), which 'kicks' in once the events of an MI start. The increased activity of the ANS is also likely to cause an increase in respiration rate. This increased rate of breathing may also be compounded by the backflow of blood to the lungs as the heart muscle starts becoming impaired and its pumping action becomes less effective.

If the individual's heart STOPS beating or beats ineffectively and therefore stops pumping blood around the body as a result of the heart muscle damage and lack of oxygen supply, resulting in disruption to the electrical conduction to the heart, then this is called a CARDIAC ARREST. Normal breathing also ceases when this occurs. For clarification, an MI is considered a circulatory (plumbing) problem, whilst a cardiac arrest is considered an electrical (wiring) problem.

People experiencing a cardiac arrest require cardiopulmonary resuscitation (CPR). CPR artificially restores oxygenated blood flow to someone whose heart has stopped beating effectively. The main components of the procedure include **chest compressions, oxygenation** (via rescue breaths i.e. 'the kiss of life' or use of appropriate device such as a face mask or ventilation device) and **defibrillation** using a defibrillator. Chest compressions, at a universally recommended rate, for example, following the rhythm of "Staying Alive" by the Bee Gees, on the sternum, compress the heart between the sternum and the thoracic spine. This allows for artificial pumping and circulation of blood to perfuse the brain and other vital organs including the heart itself and gives the individual a chance at being resuscitated. Thank God, I did not have a cardiac arrest . . . my fearfully and wonderfully made precious little heart kept pumping and DID NOT STOP!

Anyone can perform CPR! The skills involved are acquired by doing a simple training course by an accredited trainer/ organisation. This may be done in a face to face session or even via an on-line training video such as the British Heart Foundation (BHF) **'CALL, PUSH, RESCUE'** videos. BHF also provides the Heart Start training schemes free of cost across the UK. Learning to perform **CPR**—**C**all for an ambulance; **P**ush on the chest; perform **R**escue breaths, may be the most important skill you learn as you may end up saving someone's life!

You may only be able, or feel comfortable to do chest compressions +/- the 'kiss of life' but even chest compressions on their own is better than doing nothing. Defibrillation can only be administered if a defibrillator is available and there is an <u>able</u> operator. However, studies have shown that there is a better chance of recovery if this is administered when it is indicated. Contrary to popular belief, a defibrillator does not restart one's heart but rather, stops it fibrillating (quivering), that is, getting it out of an abnormal ineffective rhythm, shocking it back into a normal effective rhythm and giving it the chance to commence beating normally to supply the body with blood and oxygen. It is worth noting where defibrillators are located in public places. In the UK, they are available to the public in busy locations like shopping centres, sports stadiums, community centres, parks and railway stations. The defibrillators in public places are automated (work using automatic settings) and are simple and safe to use. They are programmed not to shock unless it is appropriate.

Research has shown that the person/s most likely to administer initial resuscitation is a relative or friend. Even if you happen to be a bystander when someone has a cardiac arrest, the initiation of CPR before the arrival of the paramedics on the scene may mean the difference between someone surviving or dying, even if it is compression only CPR.

Statistics have shown that a victim's chance of survival may be doubled in some cases if a bystander initiates CPR including defibrillation before the emergency team arrives. The survival rate is around 11% if bystander CPR is not in place (find more information at my website www. fearfullyandwonderfully.org).

As I began to experience all the ANS symptoms described earlier, I felt more unwell and on the verge of collapsing. *"Where is the ambulance? It's beginning to feel like ages!"* I managed to dial 999—*"Better two calls than one"* I thought—knowing that Tracey had already called. I relayed my signs and symptoms, telling the female call-handler that I was a doctor, that it was "my heart" and that I felt I was about to collapse! By this point my speech was barely audible. She kindly remained on the phone with me until the ambulance arrived.

The three paramedics didn't exactly spring into 'ACTION' as I envisioned! When they arrived they seemed just a bit 'less urgent' than I anticipated. Perhaps my brain was in overdrive and expecting too much, or was I just being a doctor conceptualising the management of an emergency—a heart attack? Despite their pleasant demeanour, there just didn't appear to be enough action, even for me with a generally laid-back disposition. Furthermore, the crew spent what seemed like precious minutes trying to get me, in my disoriented state, to secure my car before walking me to the ambulance. To this day, I am not sure how I managed to accomplish both these activities given the state I was in!

It soon became apparent that the ambulance crew did not quite share the urgency of my problem. The senior paramedic asserted, with words to the effect of: "Oh dear! Another GP thinking the worst! Why do you doctors always think you are having a heart attack?" My attempts to impress upon the crew the urgency to get me to the specialist cardiac hospital at Glenfield were futile and I did not have much fight left in me by that time. The verdict after their conversation with the staff at Glenfield was: "take her to the LRI A&E for blood test".

My electrocardiogram (ECG)—'heart tracing' was not showing the classic signs of a heart attack at the time, rather the readings were apparently interpreted as 'peaked T waves' or 'high take off'. Coupled with the fact that I was classified as a young female with no apparent risk factors for coronary heart disease (CHD), I feel my case was not treated as the emergency it actually was. I was very disappointed at being transported to the LRI when I felt I was having a heart attack and needed to go to the Glenfield. *Was I wrong? What was happening to me? This is certainly not right! I know my body and I have never been this ill!" "Anyway, I will be a good patient and allow these professionals to do their job,"*—I told myself!

Despite the uncertainties at the time surrounding my diagnosis, the ambulance crew commenced treating me as a case of Acute Coronary Syndrome (ACS)—a terminology used for diseases of the heart resulting from ischaemia (lack of blood supply) to the heart muscles. This usually results in one of three conditions, namely: Unstable Angina (chest pain even at rest) and either of two types of heart attack, which we doctors refer to as NSTEMI (less severe but still serious and more common. It is a **partial blockage** of one or more coronary arteries) or STEMI (the more serious of the two types. STEMI occurs when there is **total blockage** of a coronary artery). Both result in serious damage to the heart muscle and are EMERGENCIES!

As such, I was given 300 mg of aspirin to chew to prevent blood clot forming in the coronary (heart) blood vessels, which could lead to complete blockage of the vessel. This is very important and is one of the first recommended actions to take if one suspects the onset of a heart attack and has no reason not to take aspirin e.g. allergies or exceeding consumption limits. I was also given Glycerine trinitrate (GTN) spray underneath my tongue to dilate (open up) the blood vessels, thereby increasing blood flow to the heart muscles. (Unfortunately, this did not relieve my chest pain, perhaps because there was already a total blockage in one of my coronary arteries). Intravenous (IV) morphine was also administered to relieve my chest pain which by now had escalated to a pain score of 10 out of 10; as well as IV ondansetron which is an antiemetic (anti-sickness medication) to counteract the side effects of the morphine, which would have compounded the already existing nausea as an ANS manifestation of the ongoing cardiac event. As a result, by the time I arrived in A&E, my pain score was about 2/10 and I felt more comfortable apart from the persistent nausea and feeling generally unwell, which were side effects of the morphine as well as the ongoing MI that my body was desperately trying to cope with.

CHAPTER 3

Accident And Emergency Department

During the hand over report to the A&E Nurse, I was once again the subject of flippant comments about a doctor thinking she is having a heart attack. The nurse remarked "well it's not cardiac" on hearing that I had not responded to the GTN spray in the ambulance.

If an individual's chest pain is caused by ischaemia from a partially blocked artery, as is the case in angina (properly called Angina Pectoris—chest pain with exertion), then the GTN will relieve the pain when it opens-up the blood vessel and allows increased blood flow to the heart muscle. If, however, there is a total blockage as is sometimes the case in a heart attack, the GTN spray will not relieve the pain and the pain will persist. The persistence of the pain in this case means either the patient is having a heart attack, or the pain is not caused by problems related to the heart. In such a scenario, the clinician's duty is to ascertain which is the most feasible, based on the patient's history (story) and investigations such as ECG and blood test, rather than to simply conclude that the pain is not of cardiac origin, that is, caused by an ischaemic heart problem. A common advice given by doctors to patients with known CHD is to use their GTN spray (or tablet) if/when they get chest pain and to presume they are having a heart attack and dial 999 if there is no relief from the chest pain after resting and using the GTN on 2 occasions, allowing five minutes between doses for the GTN to have its effect. As such, individuals who suffer from CHD, whether or not they have had an MI should always carry their GTN spray/tablet on their person.

Shortly after arriving in A&E, I had a sample of blood taken for the relevant blood tests and also had an X-ray done. I soon learnt that my blood troponin level was raised to >250ng/l on the initial blood test. (The hospital lab measures **Troponin I** against a reference of <5ng/l to rule out an MI— taking the patient's history i.e. the patient's story, including time of onset of chest pain into consideration. NB: Troponin levels may be measured as **Troponin I** or **Troponin T**.)

This high troponin blood level concerned me as an indication that my heart muscle was being damaged causing these specific proteins (troponins) to leak into my systemic circulation. Troponin is specific to the heart muscle; it is released when there is damage to the heart muscle usually from a heart attack. Troponin may also be raised in other conditions that cause damage to the heart muscles, e.g. a pulmonary embolism (blood clot in the lungs) or other chronic conditions, e.g. heart failure or chronic kidney disease. It is, therefore, worth noting that the interpretation of troponin blood levels must not be done in isolation but in the context of a patient's clinical presentation. The NICE guidelines (CG95) 2016 alludes to this as does the World Health Organisation's (WHO) universal definition of MI (see accompanying website www.fearfullyandwonderfully. org).

Given the nature of my clinical presentation, and the fact that I was previously well, there was only one logical conclusion to make regarding the raised level of troponin in my blood—my heart muscle was leaking troponin as a result of an ischaemic event—a heart attack! The question is: Is this an NSTEMI or a STEMI, that is, is this heart attack caused by a partial or full blockage to my coronary artery/arteries?

My chest x-ray did not show any signs of chronic lung or heart problems. This suggests there were no longstanding problems, which may have resulted in enlargement of my heart (cardiomegaly), which would show on a chest x-ray.

I also understood that there were dynamic changes on my ECG, i.e. though the initial ECG was inconclusive, the subsequent ECGs done in A&E were beginning to show changes more consistent with a heart attack.

Unfortunately, despite these findings and changes as well as a further rise in my blood troponin levels to >600 ng/l indicating ongoing cardiac muscle damage, no doctor came to speak to me regarding my clinical status, a provisional or confirmed diagnosis and my management plan, including any plans to transfer me to the GH. This, despite my requests on several occasions to speak to a medical colleague. Moreover, my chest pain resurged following my admission to the A&E and I was also plagued with significant nausea and vomiting throughout despite repeated doses of antiemetics.

I explained to the nurses that I did not feel able to cope with further doses of morphine injections after a 3rd dose. Other analgesics (pain relieving medicines) were administered but unfortunately, my chest pain persisted.

When a medical colleague eventually came to speak to me, I was duly told that there were a certain number of patients in A&E and each, including me had to wait their turn. Furthermore, there were a number of patients specifically waiting for a bed at GH.

"Was this delay happening as a direct result of the staff and resource shortages in the NHS (National Health Service)? After all, it was 22nd January, still in the depths of a British winter! Could this be a consequence of the much talked about NHS winter crisis? Were there other factors at play here? Whatever, it was, that moment was a very sad one for me. At that point, the ongoing assault to my physical heart was secondary. I felt a different kind of pain in my 'heart', an emotional pain—I couldn't believe what I was hearing from my colleague and what I was experiencing in the same institution that I have served for years! Certainly, any patient with clear evidence of a heart attack needs and MUST RECEIVE priority treatment, regardless of who they are!! Keeping a patient and their loved ones informed is integral to good management, particularly in such a traumatic and frightening situation.

I choose to detail the events in A&E in order to highlight certain aspects of and deficiencies within our health care system. Our precious NHS is at risk of failing patients! Being a doctor did not make a difference and did not help my cause at this crucial time in my life. In fact, I felt that I was being directly discriminated against for being a doctor. It was as if being a doctor hampered my management! I thought about the many unpaid hours I worked as a junior doctor in the NHS, just making sure that a patient's management was left in a safe state before daring to leave for home, or on occasions, time spent talking to patients and their family members or carers just to provide some explanation and/or reassurance about their condition and care. Sadly, no one appeared to be reciprocating that action when I needed it.

In England, doctors are not given any 'perks' when they need to use the NHS. Moreover, most doctors are cognizant of being seen to make a fuss and many often keep quiet even when it is apparent that they themselves or their loved ones are not receiving the most appropriate or effective treatment (at least two colleagues have confessed this to me after hearing about my experience). This was exactly the scenario being played out in my case in A&E. Moreover, I did not wish for my husband to intervene for the same reason of not wanting to be seen to cause a fuss.

It is true that I had access to resources including senior medical colleagues that I could have called and requested their intervention. However, I chose not to, but rather to be a 'normal patient'—accessing the same resources that everyone else is entitled to access. Was this the correct thing to do? Bearing in mind, my judgement was clouded at the time and I genuinely expected that the NHS would take good care of me when I needed it!

Even if one could afford it, there are no private emergency (A&E) departments in England (though there are some private ambulance services). Whether or not one has the resources to pay for private treatment, the same NHS emergency departments are used for everyone.

So, should the doctors whom patients rely upon for their care be given some preferential treatment when using the NHS? Therein lies a topic for debate ... The impact on NHS services of a GP being off sick for a protracted period in a resource strapped NHS bears thinking about. Would doctors, patients and HR departments stand to benefit if the NHS helps the doctor as a matter of priority in the first place? What would the Great British public think? Or rather, how would the tabloids report this?

Needless to say, this experience has prompted me to perform a deep introspection and to reflect again on my own practice as a doctor. I am aware that we are currently undergoing very difficult times in the NHS, primarily due to staff shortages and it is true that chest pains can be very difficult to manage. "Ruling out" or "ruling in" a heart attack and moreover, an NSTEMI versus a STEMI, is often a diagnostic feat because patients' presentations are often non-specific and are not simply black and white. However, in this case, the clinical presentation, examination, observation and investigation findings and ongoing chest pains provided ample evidence that this said patient (who happened to be me) was experiencing a heart attack that was not letting up!

As part of my reflection, I wanted to find out whether my experience was a rarity. Unfortunately, there is evidence to indicate that women suffer disproportionately in comparison to men regarding misdiagnoses of MIs. This does not just apply to the UK as similar statistics have emerged from studies conducted in the USA, Spain and Sweden (see www. fearfullyandwonderfully.org).

The following is a quote from an article found on the British Heart Foundation (BHF) website:

> **"Despite 28,000 women dying of a heart attack in the UK each year, a study has shown that women had a fifty percent higher chance than men of receiving the wrong initial diagnosis following a heart attack. Like men, some women also often fail to recognise the signs and symptoms of a heart attack".**

The article describes the account of a 49-year-old experienced nurse who had a heart attack on her way to work.

She expressed how she didn't realise what was happening to her. Two days later the pain became excruciating and spread to her jaw, so her sister made her call an ambulance.

She recalled, "When the paramedics arrived they told me I was just having a panic attack, so I was taken to the hospital with no urgency". It was only when she was seen hours later that she was diagnosed as having had a heart attack.

She stated, "Knowing how much this delayed diagnosis could have put my life at risk, I wish I'd recognised the symptoms and called the ambulance immediately. It's so important to act fast and get the medical help you need. I'm now more aware that heart disease can affect anyone at any time—but at the time a heart attack was the last thing I thought could be happening to me".

The BHF further states that this UK study carried out by researchers from the University of Leeds showed a higher misdiagnosis for women. The research used the heart attack register of England, Wales and Northern Ireland, MINAP— **The Myocardial Ischaemia National Audit Project** and found that overall; almost <u>one-third</u> of patients had an initial diagnosis which differed from their final diagnosis.

Furthermore, the research found that women who had a final diagnosis of STEMI had a <u>59 percent</u> greater chance of misdiagnosis compared with men. Women who had a final diagnosis of NSTEMI had a <u>41 percent</u> greater chance of an MI Misdiagnosis when compared with men.

The research also reports that an average of 77 women die of a heart attack per day! At present, there are around 275,000 female heart attack survivors living in the UK—many of whom will be living with heart failure as a consequence of their heart attack. <u>The longer a heart attack is left undiagnosed and untreated, the more the heart muscle can be irreversibly damaged.</u>

Dr Chris Gale, Associate Professor of Cardiovascular Health Sciences and Honorary Consultant Cardiologist at the University of Leeds who worked on the study, said: "We need to work harder to shift the perception that heart attacks only affect a certain type of person. Typically, when we think of a person with a heart attack, we envisage a middle-aged man who is overweight, has diabetes and smokes. This is not always the case; heart attacks affect the wider spectrum of the population—including women."

Unfortunately, in my case, despite recognising the signs and symptoms of an MI and calling for help early, there was still significant delay in my diagnosis and receiving appropriate management. It appears that these phenotypical mis-perceptions, which are held by the general public as well as health care professionals, the reasons for their prevalence and how this impacts patient care, are areas that also require further research.

It is worth noting that one of the reasons why heart attacks are perceived to be more of a male's disease and less expected in women, particularly younger women, is the fact that women are protected somewhat by the hormone oestrogen during our pre-menopausal years. This means that a women's risk of getting a heart attack rises after the menopause. However, HRT is not recommended as treatment for prevention of heart attacks.

All the above alludes to the fact that both women and health care professionals need to be more alert to these facts and women need to have a heightened awareness of the signs and symptoms of a heart attack, which may not be a typical or classic presentation.

CHAPTER 4

Glenfield Hospital/
Coronary Care Unit

I was eventually transferred to the GH around 4am the following morning, at least 14 hrs after I first arrived in A&E with a heart attack. At GH, I was given further analgesics and antiemetics, therefore, began to feel better. The senior cardiologist on duty (Cardiology Specialist Registrar— Trainee cardiologist just below consultant level) had a conversation with me shortly after my arrival and provided an update on their examination findings and test results. He confirmed that I had suffered an MI; most likely an evolving STEMI (my final diagnosis at discharge was an Anterior STEMI).

I was taken to the cardiac catheter laboratory later that morning and had a coronary angiogram which confirmed total blockage to one of my major coronary arteries—the Left Anterior Descending (LAD) artery requiring percutaneous coronary intervention (PCI) also called coronary angioplasty, that is, the insertion of a stent, which is a short tube of stainless steel mesh into my LAD artery. This is expected to remain in place for life (stents are not usually replaced) but I will take additional medication (Ticagrelor) for a year specifically to protect my stent by further reducing the possibility of clot formation.

Other treatments for blocked coronary artery/arteries include thrombolysis using special 'clot busting drugs' or open-heart coronary bypass surgery using blood vessels from other parts of the body to replace the damaged coronary artery/arteries, called Coronary Artery Bypass Graft referred to as CABG. In January 2017, MINAP reported that PCI has been established as best practice for re-opening the blocked arteries that cause a heart attack. Nine out of ten patients that suffer an MI in England, receive PCI treatment.

I have not had any further chest pain since the PCI and stent insertion, indicating good revascularisation (re-establishment of the blood supply to the heart muscles). Thank God! This is also testament to the highly skilled work done by the excellent cardiology team that attended to me at GH.

Unfortunately, the ultrasound scan of my heart—Echocar-diogram (ECHO) done subsequently, revealed significant damage to my left ventricular heart muscles resulting in severe Left Ventricular Systolic Dysfunction (LVSD) with an ejection fraction of around 18%! The ejection fraction is a measure of the heart's 'squeezability'. The heart's ability to squeeze out 60-75% of the total amount of blood in its ventricles is deemed enough to perfuse all the body's tissues and is considered normal. An ejection fraction of 18% is severely reduced and is potentially life-changing for a previously well

49-year-old active person. This indicates a diagnosis of Heart Failure. However, my clinical signs and symptoms will be considered more important than the percentage of my ejection fraction. Furthermore, I have every faith that this will improve with time especially as I anticipate a miraculous healing of my heart!

In addition to the coronary angiogram and ECHO done in hospital, I also had further blood tests and another chest x-ray. Repeated ECGs were also taken to detect any changes in the electrical activity of my heart; in fact, I was kept connected to a heart monitor for the first few days in order for my heart to be constantly monitored for any such problem. The monitor also allowed for my blood pressure and heart rate to be constantly monitored as well as for easy measurement of my oxygen saturation levels by attaching the relevant probe when needed. Heart rhythm problems (arrhythmias) often occur following a heart attack due to damage caused to the 'electrical wiring' of the heart secondary to the heart muscle damage.

During my hospital stay, I also had discussions with the cardiologists about having an Implantable Cardioverter Defibrillator (ICD). I have been screened for the Subcutaneous (under the skin) ICD (S-ICD) and passed the screening, hence, I would be a suitable candidate for this type of ICD if it is deemed necessary. An ICD is made up of two parts:

1. A pulse generator—the ICD box and
2. one, two or three electrode leads.

The ICD box is slightly bigger than a small matchbox, weighing about 3 ounces. It contains an electronic circuit which is powered by a lithium battery, in a sealed metal unit.

In addition to the above tests, monitoring and screening I also had repeated physical examinations, e.g. listening to (auscultating) my chest to identify problems such as any new arrhythmias, new heart murmurs or collection of fluid in my lungs, checking my ankles for swelling and just to check how I appeared generally and how I was mentally and emotionally.

I was also commenced on several medications usually used for treating individuals after an MI. Medical science advocates that I will need to continue on most of these medicines for the rest of my life! The main reasons for the medications are to:

- Help prevent another heart attack.

- Protect the stent that I have in my Left Anterior Descending (LAD) coronary artery.

- Help to reduce the risk factors for CHD, such as reducing my cholesterol even further and to control blood pressure if indicated.

- To help to strengthen the pumping action of my heart.

- To prevent (or treat) the symptoms of angina.

I have also been commenced on medications for Heart Failure (HF) as a result of the significant damage to my left ventricular muscle and am under the Heart Failure Team which will also review me in the community- outside of hospital.

In addition to the HF team, I will also be followed up by the cardiology team in the hospital's outpatient clinics, the cardiac rehabilitation team and perhaps, the cardiac rhythm team especially if I do require an S-ICD. My follow-up plans include a repeat ECHO to be done 3 months after the initial scan.

I was very happy to be discharged from hospital after 5 days. Though I was keen to be out, I was mindful of the importance of remaining in hospital until the cardiology team was happy that it was safe for me to be discharged home. The effects of an MI on anyone's body is massive and this is compounded by the actions of the new medications which require monitoring and titration (balancing maximum effectiveness with side effects) to get to the most effective dose for each individual. It is also integral to your chance of maximum recovery that all the planned outpatients and community appointments are clear and even if appointment dates are not given prior to being discharged, one must know how these will be communicated and within what timeframe—reducing anxiety and allowing for you to take action, e.g. making relevant telephone calls if necessary. It is also paramount to take time to learn about the various medications and ensure you leave the hospital with an adequate supply to last until your own GP is able to commence supplying the repeat medications.

CHAPTER 5

Risk Factors For Myocardial Infarction

A risk factor is anything that increases one's chance of getting a disease. As I listed in my thoughts earlier, I do not have any of the conventional risk factors that are associated with CHD. In fact, when my risk of getting an MI was calculated using the risk calculators (Q-risk preceding my heart attack and BHF Heart age Calculator after my heart attack), using the same pre-MI parameters, the results indicated that I was at a low risk of getting an MI or stroke, advising that my parameters showed that I could expect to live into my 80s without having an MI/stroke. This is not to say that the risk calculators are useless but, in my opinion, are highlighting the fact that some unknown parameters may not be accounted for in these risk calculators, essentially warranting further research in this area. However, these calculators at least, provide a guideline to inform us and to prompt necessary lifestyle changes if nothing else.

As such, for me the heart attack was a reminder of the fact and my very strongly held belief that I was never an accident or a chance occurrence on this earth! Neither was this event! I believe that every human being who has graced the face of this earth has a role and purpose which fits perfectly in God's grand scheme of things, even if not immediately understood or welcomed! Hence, I aspire to do as the Bible verse taken from 1 Thessalonians 5:18 King James Version (KJV) encourages—"In everything give thanks: for this is the will of God in Christ Jesus concerning you." The counsel is to give thanks **IN** all things, not **FOR** all things!

A heart attack/MI usually occurs as a result of disease to the arteries supplying the heart muscles, known as coronary arteries (more on these later). In this condition, fatty deposits called atheroma in the lumen (cavity/bore) of the artery walls cause narrowing of the inside of the arteries which restrict blood flow. The areas of fatty deposits in the arteries' lumen are called plaques. The plaques are fragile and are more easily cracked/damaged than the normal layer covering or lining the walls of the artery. Even the movements caused by normal blood cells may cause the plaque to rupture (crack/burst). Once there is a rupture in the plaque for whatever reason, the body will naturally try to repair the damage by forming a blood clot to repair the damaged plaque. In any other area of the body, such a blood clot would be a welcome solution to a damaged and bleeding body tissue but in the already narrowed coronary artery, this can be disastrous—causing further narrowing to the lumen of the artery and eventually blockage, cutting off the blood supply to the muscle of the heart resulting in no oxygen and eventual death to that part of the heart (NB: The aspirin given when an MI is suspected is to prevent/reduce the formation of such a blood clot).

Atheroma and subsequent plaque formation is usually caused by factors which render the coronary arteries susceptible to damage. These include lifestyle practices such as smoking, increased alcohol intake, poor dietary choices such as increased saturated fats, sugars and reduced amount of fibre in the diet from fruits and vegetables.

Being overweight, which is often a result of poor diet and reduced exercise is also a risk factor. One's age (increased over 65 years), gender (higher in males) and ethnicity (higher incidence in Black and Minority Ethnic groups in the UK) are also risk factors as are existing chronic diseases, such as Hypertension and diabetes mellitus. Another factor that is important is genetic disease or familial risk factors such as a family history of CHD e.g. from a condition called familial hypercholesterolaemia (FH).

Other inherited conditions which may cause an MI include inherited abnormal heart rhythms, such as Long QT Syndrome (LQTS); Short QT Syndrome (SQTS); Brugada Syndrome; or Progressive Cardiac Conduction Defect (PCCD). For more information on these and other medical terms/symptoms mentioned, see www. fearfullyandwonderfully.org. All these conditions may lead to 'Sudden Arrhythmic Death Syndrome' (SADS). There are also the cardiomyopathies, which may be inherited and cause sudden cardiac death. Cardiomyopathy is a disease of the heart muscle which affects its size, shape and structure. This would have been one of the conditions that the doctors were looking for when they took my x-rays in A&E, along with the ECHO performed at GH.

Common cardiomyopathies include hypertrophic cardiomyopathy (HOCM) and dilated cardiomyopathy. These conditions are often the cause when a fit young athlete such as a footballer collapses and dies suddenly on the pitch. The changes that occur to one's heart **are different for each type of cardiomyopathy and can affect people differently.** However, the common pathology is that the cardiomyopathies all affect the structure of the heart and reduce its ability to pump blood around the body. They may also affect the way the heart's electrical system causes the heart to beat.

Since my MI, I have learnt that my maternal grandfather died of a heart attack at the age of 46. However, I have no further information and I'm unable to ascertain/deduce whether he suffered with an arrhythmic problem or a cardiomyopathy. It is unlikely that his cardiac disease was as a result of FH. I am not aware that he has any 1st degree relative (children) who suffered from significant hypercholesterolaemia (high blood cholesterol) or, indeed, a sudden cardiac event including an MI. Even as a 2nd degree relative (grandchild), my total cholesterol level was 4.7 mmol/l which is within normal range. As GPs we generally encourage patients to aim for a total cholesterol level below 5 (unless in special circumstances when it is beneficial to be significantly lower).

There is the remote possibility that I have some kind of unknown genetic disorder which renders my blood vessels more susceptible to injury than the normal population. Such a condition could lead to increased inflammatory risk, eventually resulting in an atherosclerotic plaque. To identify and understand this condition would require some unusual investigations, including special blood tests.

At this point, the only other factor for me to consider in my case is that of stress. Stress is now considered an independent risk factor for CHD in the following scenarios:

1. Takotsubo Syndrome (also called Broken Heart Syndrome), causes MI as well as a transient HF.

Takotsubo Syndrome is somewhat of an enigmatic disease which is still the subject of much scientific research. It usually occurs in people who have experienced intense emotional or physical stress. But in some cases there is no identifiable trigger. The exact cause is unknown but one theory is that exposure to an emotionally traumatic event causes a surge of adrenaline at levels that are harmful to the heart, causing the heart muscle to become suddenly weakened or 'stunned' and the left ventricle changes shape affecting the heart's ability to pump blood.

The initial presentation of Takotsubo Syndrome is similar to that of a heart attack including chest pain, breathlessness or collapse. There are also ECG changes and blood test results mimicking a heart attack, the difference being that when doctors examine the coronary arteries via a coronary angiogram, there will be no evidence of blockages as would be present after a heart attack. Instead, doctors will see that the heart muscle is not working properly, and the left ventricle of the heart is larger than normal.

Such findings would prompt the cardiologist to ask the patient about any recent stressful event that may have triggered the acute attack.

2. A study in 2013 showed that a genetic trait known to make people sensitive to stress also appears to be responsible for an increased risk of heart attack or death in heart patients. Researchers focused on a genetic variation that causes a hyperactive reaction to stress.

Patients with this genetic variation were found to have the highest rates of MIs and deaths. Even after adjusting for age, obesity, smoking history and other risk factors, the genetic trait was associated with an increased heart disease risk.

BHF Associate Medical Director, Professor Jeremy Pearson, said of the above: "These interesting results provide further evidence that stress may directly increase heart disease risk.

"By finding a possible mechanism behind this relationship (between stress and heart disease), these researchers have suggested tackling the problem either by changing behaviour or, if needed, with existing medicines."

3. Furthermore, according to research presented at the British Cardiovascular Society (BCS) Conference in Manchester, June 2016, mental stress could put heart disease patients at increased risk of a dangerous event, such as a heart attack. Though this is not applicable to me personally as I did not suffer with a pre-existing cardiac disease, it proves the impact of stress on serious cardiac events. Under acute mental stress, the researchers saw an increased inability of the blood

to flow through the small blood vessels in the heart resulting in an inability to supply the increased demand for blood supply and oxygen to the heart muscle.

4. Recent research from Harvard Medical School, published in the Lancet, showed that patients with heightened activity in the amygdala, a region of the brain involved in stress, could be at greater risk of heart disease and stroke.

5. Stress as an independent risk factor for MI, not only manifests as the acute stress reaction seen in Broken Heart Syndrome, but as a result of a specific genetic trait, association with heightened activity in the amygdala of the brain and also as a consequence of the protracted effects of stress over a prolonged period. This effect may be seen in individuals who have highly stressed jobs, display a certain personality type or are subjected to sustained stressful situations for other reasons. In this scenario, it is postulated that stress may cause MIs by subjecting the coronary blood vessels to the effects of increased stress hormones including cortisol and adrenaline for prolonged periods causing an inflammatory response and subsequently atherosclerosis and plaque formation.

Previously, the link between stress and increased risk of developing heart disease focused on the lifestyle habits people take up when they feel stressed such as smoking, drinking too much alcohol and overeating. However, whilst more research is needed, these studies are shedding new light on risk factors for CHD. Smoking, high blood pressure and diabetes are well-known risk factors, but the research suggests the possibility of a direct link between stress levels and heart disease.

Exploring the brain's management of stress and discovering why it increases the risk of heart disease, will shed additional light on this area of risk for CHD and allows us to develop new ways of managing chronic psychological stress.

This could lead to ensuring that individuals who are at risk are routinely screened, perhaps including 'stress' as a parameter in CVD risk calculators and to ensure that their stress is managed effectively. Including stress as a risk calculator parameter would require much research, for example, one question to be answered would be how can the level of stress in an individual be quantified?

It is hoped that the findings may be a starting point in finding new ways to target and treat stress-related heart and circulatory disease.

CHAPTER 6

Complications Of Myocardial Infarction

As stated earlier, one possible immediate complication of an MI is cardiac arrest and subsequent death, if the heart function is not restored in a timely manner! I am grateful that my heart did not stop; neither did I experience any cardiac arrhythmias. I believe that I was spared from death by my creator because He still has work for me to do on this earth. Like the biblical King David, I proclaim, "I shall not die but live and declare the works of the Lord." (KJV, Psalm 118:17). Perhaps I was spared in order to tell my story and reach individuals in an unconventional way. Whatever the reason, I regard myself as having 'work' to do before my time on this earth is completed.

The other perspective I take is that my survival chances were improved because I employed good lifestyle practices over the years, including never smoking, taking regular exercise which strengthened my heart muscles, so they were able to withstand the significant insult and continued to pump! This is purely anecdotal, but a good foundation/starting point is always a strength. More so, being in good general health allows for quicker and optimum recovery from any illness. This includes one's emotional and psychological recovery.

An MI always causes some permanent damage to the heart muscle. However, the sooner treatment is received, the more muscle it is possible to save. Unfortunately, unlike other body tissues e.g. skin or bone, heart muscle cells (cardiomyocytes) do not regenerate once damaged, unless a miracle occurs! Some remodelling of the heart's tissue occurs, however, a type of scar tissue is formed, rather than a replacement of the original muscle. Therefore, there is suboptimal functioning, including that of the heart muscle's contractility.

Heart failure will result if there is extensive damage to the cardiac muscles resulting from the lack of blood supply and oxygen to the tissues. This affects the pumping action of the heart. This is manifested as extensive breathlessness, swollen ankles which may extend to the legs in more severe cases, tiredness and reduced ability to carry out day-to-day activities. According to the BHF, for patients diagnosed with **severe** heart failure, the chances of surviving for more than five years are worse than most forms of cancer. I mention this not for scaremongering but to highlight the serious nature of this condition, which is potentially preventable.

Some people get/continue to get ANGINA especially with exertion after receiving treatment for an MI as there is still narrowing of one or more of the coronary arteries. The coronary angiogram did not identify extensive disease in my coronary arteries; hence, there was no requirement for surgical intervention, such as a coronary artery bypass graft (CABG).

The insertion of the stent to my LAD (Left Anterior Descending) artery was deemed to be enough in my case. It appears to be working well, maintaining patency in my LAD artery and allowing good blood flow to the cardiac muscles which it serves, especially as I have not experienced any angina. Thank God and thanks also to the very skilled cardiologist and cardiac team involved in performing this wonderful procedure!

In essence, the complications after an MI occur as a result of decreased contractility (reduced pumping ability); electrical instability; and tissue necrosis (death of tissues). By way of further explanation:

- **Decreased contractility** is the mechanism responsible for resulting heart failure and may also result in dangerously low blood pressure and ischaemia of the rest of the heart tissue/muscles, which can cause a serious condition called cardiogenic shock. Another consequence of decreased contractility is a predisposition to thrombus (clot) formation as a result of the sluggish blood flow/stagnation in the left ventricle. If a piece of this clot breaks off, the resulting embolus (displaced clot) may cause a stroke or infarction (tissue death due to circulatory blood loss) to other organs leading to organ failure.

- **Electrical instability** may result in arrhythmias due to disorganised ion flows within the cardiomyocytes or disruption to the electrical conduction system within the heart. As mentioned earlier, this could lead to a cardiac arrest and sudden death.

- **Tissue necrosis,** otherwise known as tissue death, triggers inflammatory reactions which can cause inflammation of the lining of the heart called pericarditis. The necrosis may also cause a hole in the middle partition wall of the heart (Ventricular Septal Defect (VSD)) causing low oxygen levels in the blood (hypoxaemia) due to the mixing of oxygenated with deoxygenated blood in the heart. A rupture of the ventricular wall from necrosis may lead to a serious condition called cardiac tamponade. Necrosis may also cause mitral regurgitation (backflow of blood through heart valves) following damage to the heartstrings (chordae tendineae) that keep these valves in place.

Most of the above conditions are rare complications of an MI; they tend to occur during the first few weeks following a heart attack. However, I have mentioned them as they are serious and important but logical complications. It is hoped that this will further raise awareness to the serious nature of an MI even if one survives it. Hence, the key message is to prevent this potentially devastating disease as much as is possible, through early screening and healthy lifestyle practices. Furthermore, the mechanisms of injuries further highlight how wonderfully made this precious organ is and how much deliberate thought and planning our creator put into constructing this highly efficient and amazing organ.

CHAPTER 7

Structure And Function
Of The Heart

Learning anatomy at medical school was both intriguing as well as arduous. Leicester medical school allows the use of human cadavers (corpses) for dissection. I want to personally thank the many individuals who kindly donate their bodies to medical education and research. We were organised in small groups when we used the Dissection Room and each group assigned a cadaver. We fondly named our group's cadaver and referred to her using that name in conversations. Looking back, I'm hoping it was a name that she would have liked! Dissecting human cadavers allowed for visualising and interacting with human organs in addition to synthetic ones. Handling the human organs and tissues brought the experience to life, no pun intended! For me, it consolidated the fact that God's attention to the details of the human heart is extraordinary!

The gross anatomy of the heart shows it as a hollow muscular pump, about the size of one's clenched fist, located in the thoracic cavity with a lung on either side. The heart is divided into four chambers—two atria (top chambers) and two ventricles (the larger lower chambers). The left ventricle has a much larger muscular mass as it pumps blood all around the body—systemic circulation. The right ventricle pumps blood only to the lungs—pulmonary circulation.

The valves allow for a one-way flow of blood through the heart and to the major blood vessels. Deoxygenated blood from the body returns to the right atria via the inferior and superior vena cavae; flows to the right ventricle via the atria-ventricular (tricuspid) valves. The right ventricle then contracts allowing blood to be passed via the semilunar pulmonary valve to the pulmonary artery which transports it to the lungs where it is oxygenated again. The left atrium receives this oxygenated blood from the lungs via the four pulmonary veins. The blood is passed through to the left ventricle via the atria-ventricular (mitral) valve.

Following the powerful contraction with the associated twisting action of the left ventricle, the oxygenated blood is passed to the entire body via the semilunar aortic valve into the aorta, where it is distributed to all the body's organs and tissues including the brain (systemic circulation). Diagrams and animations explaining the above are available at www. fearfullyandwonderfully.org

The fibrous tissue surrounding the heart is called the PERIcardium; the contractile muscle that forms the walls and middle partition (septum) of the heart, which is thickest in the left ventricle, is called MYOcardium and the very smooth squamous cells lining the inside of the heart form the ENDOcardium.

In considering how the heart is fearfully and wonderfully made, it is worth pausing at this time to examine some fascinating features of the cardiac muscle cells (cardiomyocytes). I know! This sounds boring! But bear with me—it's really quite fascinating! I need to use the language of histology and chemistry to explain God's meticulous attention to detail, in order to show you just how perfectly your heart functions! The following are examples of cardiomyocytes unique characteristics:

- Some are branching in appearance, just a differentiating feature from other muscle cells.

- They are packed full of mitochondria (the cell's engine room) as they require a lot of energy to support the ongoing cell contractions. This causes the cardiomyocytes to be highly resistant to fatigue.

- The cardiomyocytes are connected to one another in two ways. One is via electrical links called gap junctions using electrical charges carried by sodium, potassium and calcium ions. These ions pass through channels in the junctions which allow the ions to flow from one cell to another. This is very important during waves of depolarisations which cause the contractions associated with each heartbeat, thus allowing concerted contractile activity. The second way the cardiomyocytes are connected is via structural links called desmosomes (like the couplings between two railway carriages). These enable a community of cells to work together as a functional unit, so they don't pull away from each other as they are contracting.

- Calcium is necessary for the 'squeezing' action of the heart muscles. The amount of calcium in the fluid surrounding the cardiomyocytes is not enough for maximum squeezing action of the heart. However, a special component in the cardiomyocytes allows extra calcium to be released in the cells, induced by the inflow of the calcium from outside the cell. The extra calcium allows the cardiac muscles to achieve their maximum contraction potential.

- Special proteins in the cardiomyocytes interact to confer the contractile ability of the heart muscles. Troponin (remember this special protein in the cardiac muscle?) controls the interaction of two proteins in the heart muscle—actin and myosin and along with calcium, permits muscular contraction.

- Unlike skeletal muscle cells, cardiomyocytes actions are involuntary, hence, they possess the amazing ability to pump continuously until the day we die!

The electrical activity of the heart is also very fascinating. It allows the heart to contract and relax in a precisely co-ordinated and regulated manner. Please indulge me as I explain this exquisitely made electrical system!

This electrical activity of the heart is not caused by the actions of the external nervous system but is INTRINSIC to the heart i.e. it is caused by specialised cardiac tissues in the myocardium which cause the depolarisation (contraction) and repolarisation (relaxation) of the heart muscles. The intrinsic nature of the electrical activities of the heart allows the heart to continue beating even if/when it is removed from the body!

The Sino-atrial node (SA node), located in the top of the right atria, somewhere near the entrance of the superior vena cava is the origin of the electrical activities of the heart and gives rise to the sinus rhythm (normal regular heart beat) in a healthy functioning heart. It is often referred to as the natural pacemaker of the heart and influences the other electrically active tissues in the heart, including the other significant area of electrical activity, the atrio-ventricular (AV node) which is located—you guessed it, between the atria and the ventricles.

There are preferential conduction pathways (tracts) of the heart's electrical activities from the SA node. One of the conducting pathways, the anterior pathway, takes impulses (electrical signals) across to the left atrium. The other tracts allow electrical signals to spread to the other areas of myocardium in the atria, allowing for depolarisation (contraction) of both atria in a co-ordinated fashion.

The valves of the heart are almost on a horizontal plain across the mid-section of the heart. They are made up of fibrous collagen tissue. Consequently, there is a ring of fibrous tissue along the valvular plain of the heart, essentially forming an AV ring of fibrous tissue between the atria and the ventricles. This ring of fibrous tissue is an electrical insulator; it does not conduct electricity, hence will not interfere with the impulses (electrical signals) travelling from the SA node to spread into the ventricles except via the preferential pathways, along the internodal tracts.

This means that in the normal functioning heart, impulses within the heart can only travel in one direction i.e. from the atria (via the SA node) to the ventricles via the AV node. Where this is not the case, impulses become chaotic or travel along an abnormal pathway resulting in arrhythmias or other pathological heart conditions. Such finely tuned design is for me, yet another example of our Creator's elegant design.

After a pause of about 40 milliseconds, the collected impulses from the AV node are passed to the "bundle of HIS" (AV bundle) which are then passed to the right and left bundle branches which subsequently divide into the PURKINJE fibres at the apex of the heart. These small branches are disseminated as little tracts/fibres into the myocardium of the ventricles, conducting the electrical impulses by these specialised cardiomyocytes, resulting in bilateral ventricular contractions. The synchronicity, magnitude, and direction of the electrical impulses causes an upward contractile motion of the ventricles along with a concurrent twisting action (as if wringing one's clothes to get all the water out), in order to maximise the output of blood from the ventricles towards the semilunar aortic and pulmonary valves into the aorta and pulmonary artery taking blood to the systemic and pulmonary circulation, namely, to the entire body and to the lungs.

The resumption of the electrical activity of the heart allows the heart ventricles to resume their resting state, in preparation for the next cardiac cycle, which typically repeats around 72 times per minute! This is necessary for optimum functioning of the ventricles and the heart as a whole and continues from the womb until the death. My husband (a chemical engineer) says, God, amongst many things, must also be an electrical engineer!

Furthermore, "Blood vessels are not just straight-through tubes, like water pipes, as was previously thought. Scientists at Imperial College, London, found that blood vessels have a slight twist to them i.e. they are helical. Colin Caro and Spencer Sherwin showed that the gentle corkscrewing makes the blood flow more evenly compared to straight vessels. They found that, with helical vessels, damage from turbulent flow was much less likely, especially at T-junctions. Smooth flow also encourages the production of health-promoting protective substances" [1]. Our Creator's attention to detail is extraordinary.

The heart has its own dedicated blood supply, known as the coronary circulation. These blood vessels are different from the main arteries and veins that carry away and supply blood to the systemic and pulmonary circulation described earlier. The coronary blood vessels encircle the entire surface of the heart to supply all the tissues of the heart. Coronary arteries supply blood to the heart muscle; like all other tissues in the body, the heart muscle needs oxygen-rich blood to function. Similarly, oxygen-depleted blood must be removed; the coronary veins remove deoxygenated blood with waste from the heart (these will not be discussed further in this book).

---

1   New Scientist 158(2134):19, May 16, 1998.

The coronary arteries wrap around the outside of the heart with small branches penetrating the heart muscle to bring it blood. The two main coronary arteries are the right and left main coronary arteries.

- Left Main Coronary Artery (LMCA). The left main artery supplies blood to the left side of the heart muscle (the left ventricle and left atrium). It divides into branches, namely:

    a. The Left Anterior Descending (LAD) artery which supplies blood to the front of the left side of the heart. This is the main branch to the left side of the heart and also partially supplies its septum (middle partition wall). It is sometimes referred to as "the widow maker" . . . guess why? (Yet another example of gender bias relating to heart attacks/MIs). Unfortunately, it was my LAD artery that was totally blocked. Thank God my husband has not become a widower!

    b. The circumflex artery which branches off the LMCA and encircles the heart muscle. This artery supplies blood to the outer left side and back of the heart.

- Right Coronary Artery (RCA) supplies blood to the right ventricle, the right atrium, and the SA (sinoatrial) and AV (atrioventricular) nodes, which regulate the heart rhythm. The RCA divides further into smaller branches, including the right posterior descending artery and the acute marginal artery. Together with the LAD artery, the RCA helps supply blood to the septum (middle) of the heart.

Since coronary arteries deliver blood to the heart muscle, it is clear that any coronary artery pathology (disease) can have serious implications by reducing the blood flow with oxygen and nutrients to the heart muscle. As seen in this book, this can lead to a heart attack and possibly death.

For the perfect functioning of the heart, therefore, there is the electrical activity, the valvular activity, and the myocardial activity all beautifully co-ordinated.

Remember earlier that I mentioned how the SA node fires around 90 impulses per minute? Well the parasympathetic nervous system innervates (supplies) the SA and AV nodes via the vagus nerve (10th cranial nerve) and slows down the natural sinus rhythm; otherwise the heart rate of an average person would be around 90-beats per minute. This explains why well and very fit individuals will have lower heart rates. Though the heart rate is naturally inhibited by the parasympathetic system it may also be stimulated or increased by the activity of the SYMPATHETIC nervous system in conjunction with the endocrine/hormonal system, hence, the influence by the hormone adrenaline in the fight/ flight response. This explains why stress, fear and anxiety stimulate the ANS (which comprises the Sympathetic and Parasympathetic nervous system) in a way that increases the heart rate, which in a stressful situation can go up to over 200 beats per minute!

God made our hearts to function in a purposeful and co-ordinated way from conception. The heart is the first formed organ in the developing foetus and the human heart begins to function in a unique and customised way from the time of birth. An example of this functioning at the time of birth is the automatic closing of the natural defect (hole) in the septum between the two ventricles in the heart of the new-born infant. This hole closes up at exactly the right time during the birth process to allow for the oxygenation of the blood from the lungs, which does not occur while the baby is in the womb and is receiving oxygen through the umbilical cord. If this defect is not closed automatically, as expected, then the result will be a baby with a Ventricular Septal Defect (VSD), otherwise called a 'hole in the heart'.

The heart pumps blood around the body through thousands of miles of blood vessels. The volume of blood in an adult human is about 5-6 litres. Cardiac Output (CO) refers to the total amount of blood that the heart pumps out per minute. In terms of mathematical equation, this is equal to the amount of blood pumped out with each heartbeat (stroke volume) x the number of heart beats per minute. Therefore, CO = stroke volume (SV) x Heart rate (HR).

The average adult's resting heart rate is about 70 beats per minute. The heart pumps about 70 ml of blood with each heartbeat. [CO=70x70ml=4900ml]. This means that approximately 5 litres of blood passes through an adult heart each minute, whilst at rest.

This would be equivalent to about 300 litres an hour or 3 full standard UK baths. In a lifetime of about 80 years (29,200 days), the heart beats over 2.9 billion times and pumps over 200 million litres or 82 Olympic swimming pools of blood!

As in the physical body, blood also has great significance to the Christian from a spiritual point of view. The Bible does teach that life is in the blood (Leviticus 17:11) and I am sure that everyone would agree that blood is essentially life! This is clearly apparent in our bodies as our blood performs the important functions of **transporting** important substances such as oxygen, nutrients, hormones and heat as well as removing debris and noxious gases from our system; **protection** by supplying specialised blood cells such as white blood cells to fight diseases and platelets to prevent devastating haemorrhaging and **regulation** through maintaining core body temperature, a very strict pH balance between acids and bases in our bodies and regulating water balance in the blood vessels and body tissues.

As Christians, we embrace the blood of Jesus Christ as a life-giving source, having similar functions of **transportation**, **protection**, and **regulation** on a spiritual level. It is ultimately the saving medium shed by our Lord Jesus Christ on the cross of Calvary to secure our salvation but also seen as a cleansing and healing medium for mankind.

CHAPTER 8

Management After A Myocardial Infarction

Many individuals still have a good quality of life and good health following an MI and that is exactly what I anticipate!

Post MI management will inevitably require changes especially if one enjoyed good health prior to the MI. Initial changes include taking regular medicines discussed earlier. The usual minimum 'cocktail' includes 'SAAB' i.e., **S**tatin, which is a cholesterol reducing medication, e.g. atorvastatin; **A**spirin and other anti-platelet medicines to reduce clotting, e.g. ticagrelor/clopidogrel, which in my case is primarily to protect the stent in my LAD artery. **A**ngiotensin converting enzymes inhibitors (ACEis) or **A**ngiotensin receptor blockers (ARBs) e.g., ramipril or candasartan and **B**etablockers, e.g. bisoprolol are also required as a minimum. If there is evidence of heart failure, as in my case, then there will also be additional medications.

Regular blood tests, particularly to monitor kidney function and monitoring blood pressure are very important whilst on these medications, especially during the early stages.

Lifestyle changes will become inevitable and are integral and crucial to one's management after a heart attack; perhaps even more so than drugs but definitely, as important! Even if you enjoyed good lifestyle practices prior to the MI, it is advisable that this is enhanced and maximised. Lifestyle practices that are vital include the following:

- Quitting smoking if you are a smoker. It is advisable to seek professional help to increase one's chance of success to quit.

- Limiting the amount of alcohol you drink. Small amounts of alcohol of 1-2 units/day has been shown to be cardio-protective in men >40 and women after the menopause. The current advice from the Department of Health (DOH) is that both men and women should not regularly drink more than 14 units per week (equivalent to about 1.5 bottles of wine or 5 pints of 5% lager). If you do drink as much as 14 units/week, it is recommended that this is spread over 3 days or more. It is worth noting that extra care should be taken with stronger beers, lagers and wine and with home/pub measurements which may be larger than usual.

- Eating a healthy, balanced diet including at least 5 portions of fruits and vegetables per day and 2-3 portions of oily fish per week, e.g. mackerel, herring, pilchards, sardines, salmon, or trout. See www.fearfullyandwonderfully. org for more detailed dietary information. Information surrounding a healthy diet is the subject of ongoing research and debate. It is worth discussing this with an approved health care professional if you require clarifications.

- Keeping physically active—at least 30 mins of moderately active exercise i.e. enough activity to get you slightly out of breath is encouraged. It is important that you do warm up activities prior to your main exercise followed by lighter cooling down activities after the main period of exertion.

- Exercise should be taken at least 5-times per week (the cardiac rehabilitation programme is excellent for providing guidance on the most appropriate individualised advice on exercise techniques and regimes) after a heart attack.

- Maintaining a healthy weight and body shape by practising all the above.

- Maintaining your total cholesterol level below 4mmol/L and BP below 130/80. These are usually checked by your GP and/or cardiac nurses regularly.

- Good control of blood glucose (sugar) levels if you are diagnosed with diabetes.

The BHF continues to invest in research to advance the management of cardiac diseases. The "Mending Broken Hearts Appeal" is to date, the most ambitious research programme in the fight against heart failure. BHF reports: "our researchers are making new heart cells, attempting to grow new heart muscle to replace lost muscle, and investigating whether we can switch on the genes that promote healing in the heart, looking at what potential the heart muscle has to heal itself".

The following excerpts taken from the BHF website provide an exciting glimpse into the various areas of research which the organisation is currently conducting. Any one of these may one day provide a cure for heart failure and other heart diseases!

Researchers are studying fish which can repair their own hearts.

Humans can't regenerate their damaged hearts, but zebrafish can! If part of their heart is damaged zebrafish can repair it in a matter of weeks, just as we are able to mend a broken bone. That's why our Mending Broken Hearts Appeal is funding researchers to find out what their secret is.

Using cells from veins to mend broken hearts— Paolo Madeddu

Paolo's research has led to the exciting discovery that a special type of cell in the veins of heart patients could help to mend a broken heart.

Paolo has shown that, in mice, pericyte progenitor cells can encourage new blood vessels to grow and improve heart function. All indications are that if these cells are delivered directly into the heart, they could be an effective way to strengthen and restore hearts weakened after a heart attack.

Using stem cells after a heart attack—Johannes Bargehr

Johannes commented "With this Mending Broken Hearts Appeal we're able to fully explore the potential of blood vessel cells that we've made in the lab to contribute to a working heart patch".

Institute of Developmental and Regenerative Medicine—Building for the future

We need to raise over £10 million to help build and establish a new cutting-edge research facility at the University of Oxford. BHF Professor Riley explains: "My vision is a world where heart damage is temporary and repairable. If the Institute becomes a reality, our research discoveries could trigger a revolution in cardiovascular medicine".

As you can see from these wonderfully encouraging excerpts, BHF are doing a great job to improve cardiovascular medicine! You will find links to these and other relevant BHF pages from www.fearfullyandwonderfully.org.

In the meantime, we can do our bit too, as evidence from epigenetics indicate that we can influence our genes! This is done primarily through our lifestyle choices. The discipline of epigenetics also describes how our habits can turn genes on and off making illnesses more or less likely in us and those we love. Hence the saying "We are what we eat!"

CHAPTER 9

The Psychological And Spiritual Impact Of Myocardial Infarction

If you have had an MI, how do you feel? How have the psychological, social, financial and spiritual ramifications of your MI affected who you are now? How has it impacted your relationships? Do you feel you have changed?

The impact of an MI can be 'full on' with an extremely frightening effect, especially if you previously enjoyed good health and a varied and full life up until the event. The effect is not just physical but affects us psychologically and spiritually as well. By extension, this also impacts your personal relationships, your place and function in society and of course, your financial standing. This all-encompassing effect delineates the importance of embracing holistic health as defined by the World Health Organisation (WHO) which defines health as a state of complete physical, mental and social well-being and not merely the absence of disease.

This definition acknowledges our compound and trichotomous (three-part) status as human beings as revealed in 1 Thessalonians 5:23, where Paul prays for our total preservation, stating: "Now may the God of peace Himself sanctify you **entirely**; and may your **spirit and soul and body** be preserved complete, without blame at the coming of our Lord Jesus Christ."

The Greek word for body is soma, hence somatic presentations refer to signs and symptoms that are physically exhibited by us when we are affected by a disease/condition. In the preceding chapters, I have detailed the somatic or physical presentations of an MI. Sometimes, psychological conditions are also manifested as somatic signs and symptoms, making a diagnosis more difficult.

Over 700 verses in The Bible mention the human heart. The Bible describes the heart (often referred to and used interchangeably with our soul) as having the capacity to **"feel"** emotions and desires e.g. ". . . because of the dread that your heart shall **feel** . . .". as described in Deuteronomy 28:67 (ESV). The word soul is from the Hebrew 'Naphesh' which refers to aspects of sentience that is the capacity to **feel**, **perceive** or **experience** subjectively. The soul is the essence of human beings; it is who we are; our self; our person; our individuality. The Bible tells us that man became a living soul after God "blew into his nostrils the breath of life" following his creation from the dust of the ground in Genesis 2:7 (KJV). Equally, the soul is removed at the time of physical death, as recorded in Genesis 35:18 (KJV) ". . . her soul was in departing, (for she died)".

Like the soul, the spirit is that non-physical part of us that connects/communicates with God who Himself is a spirit, as described in John 4:24 (KJV) "God is a Spirit: and they that worship Him must worship Him in spirit . . ." It therefore, allows us to <u>worship</u>, to have intuition and is said to be that part of us which **"knows"** as described by 1Corinthians 2:11 (NET) "For who among men knows the things of a man except the man's spirit within him?", thus, our **mind**, **intellect**, **will** and **conscience**. The word spirit comes from the Hebrew word Ruach, meaning wind, and the Greek word Pneuma, meaning breath, both conveying an invisible force. Many of our medical terminologies are derived from the Greek pneuma, e.g. pneumonia, pneumothorax, both of which refer to conditions involving the lungs—having to do with wind/air/breath. As humans, our spirit is therefore the element that gives us the ability to communicate and have an intimate relationship with God.

Sometimes the words soul and spirit are used interchangeably, and it is often difficult to explain the difference between the two, in fact, there are theological debates surrounding this issue. However, my own views are that though the two are connected, as both deal with the non-physical aspects of how we as humans experience this life, they are separable as described by Hebrews 4:12 (KJV) "For the word of God is quick, and powerful, and sharper than any two-edged sword, piercing even to the dividing asunder of soul and spirit . . ." Both the soul and spirit, therefore, are the centre of our psychological, emotional, social and spiritual experiences which are unmistakably impacted after an MI.

Immediately after an MI, the physical body will be trying to cope with the affliction experienced by the heart! However, as soon as one has the opportunity to ponder and assimilate the events of an MI, the realisation of what happened, the implications and questions about the event will start pouring in. The effect will, therefore impact on the individual's holistic health.

The psychological impact may include signs and symptoms of depression and or anxiety. Depression is very common after any life-changing experience. According to Professor Steptoe, Professor of Psychology at the BHF, it has become clear over the last 20 years or so that some people have quite severe psychological reactions following an MI, in particular, suffering with quite high levels of depressive symptoms. The large-scale studies conducted in the area of psychological impact of MI show both in the UK and in other countries that around 15% of people who have survived a heart attack become quite seriously depressed in the first few weeks following the event. For some, that depression will be quite persistent. Approximately another 25% experience milder levels of depressive symptoms, or anxiety symptoms; in total about 40% of patients do experience quite severe emotional responses, which have been linked with long term problems as far as their cardiovascular health is concerned, so it is a significant problem!

The BHF research has found that those who get depressive symptoms are actually more likely to have recurrent cardiac problems. For instance, it is thought that those suffering from depressive symptoms are twice as likely to have another heart attack or to die of heart disease. There is a growing concern regarding this link, how and why it exists, and what can be done to remedy it (for more information see www. fearfullyandwonderfully.org).

Signs and symptoms of depression include frequent feelings of sadness or emptiness; feelings of worthlessness or helplessness; loss of appetite or overeating/'comfort eating', poor sleeping patterns including early morning waking or sleeping excessively; fatigue; unexplained aches and pains that don't respond to treatment; difficulty concentrating or remembering; loss of interest in previously pleasurable activities or the outside world; irritability; excessive crying for no apparent reason; thoughts of suicide and death.

It is worth noting that some of these signs and symptoms may not be indicative of depression e.g. poor sleep pattern and increased lethargy may also result from poor sleep which may occur as a result of one struggling to find a suitable/comfortable sleeping position due to breathlessness. During the period following my discharge from hospital, the breathlessness caused me considerable discomfort at nights. This meant having to sleep in an upright position propped up by around 5 pillows. The V-shaped pillow I later acquired greatly assisted me in finding a more comfortable sleeping position.

In addition, there is no shame in crying occasionally after such a life-changing event—I definitely felt the need to on occasions! Crying can often be a way of releasing emotional tension. However, if this is excessive and persistent and associated with other feelings of depression, then one needs to seek professional assessment and advice. Your GP would be your first port of call in this case.

Psychological impact also includes feeling anxious and unsettled and battling with fears about the possibility of a recurrent MI or occurrence of complications.

In terms of anxiety experiences, some people find the whole experience extremely stressful and are overwhelmed with thoughts that they might be dying. This may remain pervasive, and individuals may constantly feel very anxious about their future health. After getting past this initial stage, MI survivors may relax a little, but are then forced to think about their lives in a different way e.g. your priorities may change significantly!

Many people, particularly young people who've had a heart attack, may not have known that they were at risk, so will find themselves suddenly confronted with the idea of their own mortality. This requires quite a lot of psychological adjustment. Personally, I had to face anxieties about not knowing the cause of my MI and therefore contemplating whether it was hereditary and could affect my children. Or, indeed, whether I need to be living my life in a radically different way, including changing my priorities significantly.

This generated a level of anxiety, though not in a pathological sense but has prompted me to explore/investigate/research other causes of MI including genetics and the role stress plays in causing a heart attack. As a result, my enquiries revealed varying and interesting findings worthy of further investigation and expert advice.

The experiences of depression and anxiety are rather different. In relation to a heart attack, a person who becomes anxious is more likely to become worried that the problem may recur. Hence, such individuals may become overly sensitive to signs and symptoms they experience e.g. palpitations or shortness of breath, which may result in a heightened state of anxiety and even panic! At high levels of anxiety this can be problematic and stop the MI survivor from doing day-to-day tasks, due to their heightened concern of such activities triggering an adverse effect.

Conversely, an individual with a depressive response is much more likely to become withdrawn and experience feelings of hopelessness. Their experience may include feelings that the worst is inevitable.

Some MI survivors may suffer from both conditions to varying degrees. The two conditions are managed in different ways as the issues for the patients can be very different, as discussed earlier. Psychological management examines different reactions with a view to understanding why people experience one problem more than the other and the extent to which they overlap.

Psychosocial interventions include conventional management for anxiety and depression. There should ideally be a focus on education about heart health; counselling or psychotherapy to cope with adjustment as well as dealing specifically with the signs and symptoms of anxiety and depression: stress management interventions; exercises and medications if deemed necessary & appropriate. These interventions are thought to best improve outcomes when they prompt lifestyle changes and better medical adherence.

The partners of MI survivors can be invaluable in providing support, whether or not individuals suffer from anxiety and or depression. However, experts have pointed out that the support partners offer often requires a delicate balance. It is important for a partner to be available, if and when the MI survivor wants to talk, but either party may find this a challenge for various reasons. A partner may also come across as 'over-solicitous' in the way they explore the feelings and meet the needs of their loved one. Conversely, it does not help if partners bury their head in the sand and carry-on with business as usual, whilst neglecting the obvious change in their circumstances brought about as a result of the MI.

Individuals may or may not develop depression or anxiety for various reasons which do not indicate that one person is better than the other. There are various factors: we are all wired differently; we are conditioned differently, mostly due to our environment and culture. Others may have stronger family/community networks, hence, receive better social, emotional and spiritual support.

As a Christian, I am able to deal with the psychosocial effect of my MI by standing firm on the promises of God, my heavenly father. I also know Him as Jehovah-Rapha (the Hebrew term which means "The LORD who Heals"), see Exodus 15:26 (ESV) ". . . I am the Lord, your healer". Jehovah-Rapha has the power to heal **physically**, as demonstrated in 2 Kings 5:10 (ESV) ". . . and your flesh shall be restored, and you shall be clean." He also heals **emotionally**, "The Lord is near to the brokenhearted and saves the crushed in spirit." (ESV, Psalm 34:18); **mentally**, as expressed by King Nebuchadnezzar after he experienced a 'mental breakdown'—"When that period of time was over, I, Nebuchadnezzar, lifted my eyes to heaven and my sanity returned to me. I blessed the Most

High, praising and honouring the one who lives forever" (ISV, Daniel 4:34); and finally **spiritually**, in that "He continues to forgive all your sins, he continues to heal <u>ALL</u> your diseases," (ISV, Psalm 103:3).

Furthermore, Jesus Christ demonstrated that He was 'The Great Physician' (Jehovah-Rapha in the flesh) by performing numerous miraculous healings of diverse diseases, as described in the New Testament Gospels of Matthew, Mark, Luke and John.

We are encouraged by Jesus in John 14:1, not to let our hearts become troubled. Paul also admonishes us by saying "Do not be anxious about anything, but in every situation, by prayer and petition, with thanksgiving, present your requests to God" (NIV, Philippians 4:6). Of-course, I do not expect this to be a natural response for everyone, especially those who are not familiar with the teachings of Christianity and/or have a pre-disposition to worrying excessively. However, applying the counselling of these Bible verses has realistically helped me to deal with the many challenges I faced and continue to encounter after experiencing an MI.

Moreover, there is evidence that our belief system and/or our faith have a significant impact on our actions and our state of being including our physical health. The following study reported that individuals who pray enjoy better health. Writing in JAMA Internal Medicine, Dr Tyler VanderWeele, a professor of epidemiology of the Harvard T.H. Chan School of Public Health in Boston found that women who went to church more than once per week had a 33 per cent lower risk of death during the 16-year study, compared with women who never attended church. He was quoted as saying that "part of the benefit seems to be that attending religious services increases social support, discourages smoking, decreases depression and helps people develop a more optimistic or more hopeful outlook on life."

For me, especially being a doctor and knowing what I know, the practice of positive contemplation, brought about by meditating on God's word, helps me to set aside many of the negative thoughts which may result from dwelling on the factual information that are less desirable, such as the knowledge of the possible implications and complications of an MI (described in earlier chapters). As such, the Bible admonishes us in Philippians 4:8 (KJV) "... whatsoever things are **pure** ... **lovely** ... of **good report**; if there be any **virtue**, and if there be any **praise**, think on these things".

I appreciate that many individuals may not have given much thought to the teachings of the Bible on health and may have doubts as to whether this 'God business' even has any role in our healing. However, it is a fact that our mind is the seat of our emotions and many if not all deliberate and unconscious outcomes are seeded in our minds. Being aware of this fact means that one can make a concerted effort to guard one's destiny by protecting one's thoughts. The following is a powerful quote by Frank Outlaw:

> "Watch your thoughts; for they become words.
> Watch your words; for they become actions.
> Watch your actions; for they become habits.
> Watch your habits; for they become character.
> Watch your character; for it will become your destiny".

The truth is that medical sciences and interventions, such as medications have limitations! It is therefore incumbent upon us as MI survivors to learn how to manage our health in its entirety and actively implement effective strategies and practices to complement our recovery. Herein lies the challenge! Unfortunately, a prescription for drugs is not a panacea for all ills. Furthermore, drugs invariably cause unwanted side effects.

My worldview means that I see the recent events in my life which have been dominated by my MI as an aspect of God's overall plan for my life. I believe that this has happened to me because God my father ALLOWED it and not just as an accident! Furthermore, I believe that God wants to teach me something valuable through this experience which will define and make me a stronger and better individual.

I draw from the analogy of processing precious metals e.g. gold or silver. The metal must be heated to extreme temperatures in order for the impurities to be eliminated from it. In the case of silver, the silversmith knows he/she has pure silver when his/her reflection can be seen clearly in the molten silver. Similarly, God wants His qualities to be reflected in me when others look at me. This is not to say that I will become perfect, rather others will acknowledge that I am flourishing and thriving regardless of my circumstances.

The important thing is that God will not allow us to undergo more than we are able to bear. He promised His children in 1 Corinthians 10:13 (NET) that "He will not let you be tried beyond what you are able to bear, but with the trial will also provide a way out so that you may be able to endure it". One might argue, why didn't God prevent this from happening in the first instance? I refer again to the above process of eliciting and revealing pure silver, remember, the metal must undergo the extreme temperature to attain its full beauty and potential!

Andrae Crouch, a famous American Gospel singer/song-writer, in his song entitled 'Through it All', penned the words "If I never had a problem, I wouldn't know that He could solve them . . ." We can never know our true strength unless we are tested. Equally, my husband informs me that in engineering, the purity and strength of any material, must be tested and measured before it can be used for any major construction. Life's trajectory is such that we will inevitably face some form of difficulties, obstacles or hardships.

The question is "what do we do with the lemons that life inevitably gives to us; do we complain about the tart acrid taste of the lemons or do we use them to make refreshing lemonade amongst other wonderful culinary delights?"

T D Jakes, a renowned American preacher/teacher/ transformational speaker, talks about the fact that heavy duty equipment is not necessary to demolish a chicken coop. Hence, when the devil moves in with tractors and cranes, then it must be inferred that a significant structure is at the centre of the demolition & building project!

The discourse about being fearfully and wonderfully made: The Heart of the Matter highlights the fact that as human beings we have the ability to think objectively and make important personal decisions that are not merely knee-jerk responses to our various life experiences, be they good or bad.

The 'heart' as the core of our soul and spirit, enables us to love and experience God intimately. As such, our hearts reveal our thoughts, memories, emotions, desires, conscience and self-will. Luke 6:45 (NET) tells us that "... his mouth speaks from what fills his heart". Our hearts, therefore, not only think, feel, and remember, but also choose the course of actions we take in our lives. This is especially true of individuals who have a personal relationship with the Lord Jesus, whose decisions should reflect integrity of heart.

One example of how this is demonstrated is how we deal with individuals who have wronged us or to situations that happen to us that appear to be undeserved or unfair. Do we become bitter and resentful or do we forgive and learn strategies to deal with the issues and propel ourselves forward?

A number of my friends/relatives have expressed to me how they have struggled with comprehending and accepting the recent events of me having an MI. One of my friends described how she felt angry with God and my sister expressed her struggles to accept why such an awful event should befall me, robbing me of so much including my health and by extension my quality of life, physically, mentally and financially by significantly restricting my career options/opportunities. I have explained to all who have expressed these that though I fully understand their points of views, I believe that this is all part of the work of my 'grand weaver'—The Lord Jesus and is all purposefully allowed to enable me to get to a higher dimension in this life. My friend and I hugged each other and cried as we recounted my close brush with death and tried to make sense of it all!

One of, if not the main thing, that I struggle with after this event, was my experience in the A&E department. Each time I reminisce about that period of time on January 22nd-23rd, I feel a wave of emotion that is difficult to describe, and I have had to consciously unpick and analyse what I feel and why I feel the way I do about this particular portion of my experience. As I stated earlier, it was a different kind of pain in my 'heart' when I realised the reality of what was happening to me at the time.

Despite all of this, however, I am determined to rise above all the challenges that have arisen as a result of experiencing an MI, and to forgive where I feel this is necessary, rather than permitting myself to become bitter. This does not mean that I will not talk about the issues and seek clarifications and answers where I think these are lacking—even from the Lord! He tells me in Isaiah 1:18 (KJV) to "... reason together ..." with Him. There is no guarantee that I will get all the answers I desire but that for me is not an excuse to become indifferent and to depart from my core convictions. More so, there are so many things to be grateful for in the circumstances and I have witnessed such an awesome outpouring of love and appreciation for me that I have chosen to focus on those realities instead. This in no way minimises the harsh realities that are an integral part of the experience; rather, it is about consciously choosing my response.

Of course, one needs the help of God's true 'agape' love to achieve an acceptable and beneficial way of thinking and acting. Paul in 1 Thessalonians 3:12 expressed a desire that the Lord would allow us to increase and abound in love towards one another and towards all men. The ultimate outcome is that of achieving holistic health as defined by the WHO.

Writing this book has played a key role in my recovery, assisting me in coping with all the various issues that have arisen. By writing the book, I have been compelled to think about things in a logical way; reinforce my own understanding of what my precious heart has just undergone and sift and analyse the impact the whole event has had on me and my family. In addition, it has helped me to formulate a strategy to deal with known and unknown future eventualities. This gives me a sense of peace, putting my HEART in a calm and moderated state.

In Proverbs 4:23 (KJV) a very high importance is placed on keeping our hearts pure: "Keep thy **heart** with all diligence; for out of it are the issues of life".

CHAPTER 10

Moving Forward After A Myocardial Infarction— Practical Issues

Only time will tell what THE OUTCOME WILL EVENTUALLY BE IN MY CASE. It is uncertain how my cardiac muscles will respond. Medical evidence dictates that cardiomyocytes do not regenerate from damage following an MI and the result from the ECHO showed extensive damage to my left ventricular wall, causing poor movements/pumping actions. This has generated a formal diagnosis of Heart Failure for me, one of the complications of an MI described earlier. The degree of heart failure I have is clinically mild[2] at present as I am not significantly affected restricting my physical and day-day activities.

Heart Failure is the term used to describe the scenario where the heart becomes less efficient at pumping blood to supply

---

2 NYHA Class II—New York Heart Association Functional Classification of Heart Failure

all the body tissues sufficiently and meet the demands of the body. As stated earlier, the resulting signs and symptoms of HF include excessive tiredness and fatigue, breathlessness at rest or with activities, swelling of the ankles/feet (or abdomen) due to fluid retention. Conventional medicine, therefore, dictates that there could be complications of heart failure and one should be aware that there may be progressive deterioration with time.

As discussed earlier, I have to consider the possibility that I may require the use of an Implantable Cardioverter Defibrillator (ICD). I am a suitable candidate for an S-ICD in case I require this following subsequent repeats of the echocardiogram not showing favourable results, that is an increase of my ejection fraction at least above 30% (from an initial recorded value of 18%). As a believer in God and, hence, in miracles, I am anticipating a full recovery and hoping that none of this will become necessary or at least, that the use of an S-ICD would only be prophylactic (preventive).

It is inevitable that the uncertainties of the future are likely to plague our minds and sometimes there are lurking questions of "what ifs" including the possibility of a repeat MI. The truth is that a previous MI increases the risk of a subsequent one. However, if one adheres to the lifestyle advised and takes the medications prescribed, the risk of a further MI is significantly reduced.

The cardiac rehabilitation program is reported to have helped many individuals and their families and or carers come to terms with the practicalities of this period. One of the main challenges concerns how MI survivors balance physical activities i.e. doing too much too soon vs. not doing enough, throughout this period. Unfortunately, in my experience, these services are stretched due to resource constraints, leading to their reduced availability and which may result in patients waiting for as long as 3 months after the event to access a first consultation session. Nonetheless, the cardiac rehabilitation program is a service worth accessing as part of one's recuperation following an MI.

As mentioned earlier, the heart is a muscle which, like other muscles in the body, requires physical activities to keep it in optimum health. Getting the balance right is integral to recovering well.

One of the key factors in the recovery process is that we feel we can speak openly about the lifestyle and all other issues that affect us and our family. It has been reported that as a result of being compelled to face these issues, many individuals have found that life after an MI may actually be better than before including in the area of managing family dynamics.

The question regarding my own function/ability is always luring—will I ever be able to return to work fully and function in the physical capacity that I previously did? Certainly, this has bio-psycho-social implications as detailed above.

One practical issue that I personally struggled with in the days immediately after suffering the MI was the significant shortness of breath. It was a feat to have a shower—singing concurrently was a BIG NO-NO! Much to my alarm and rude awakening to not being able to do a simple activity that I'd always taken for granted. Thank God, I am now able to sing again in the shower and even if not previously regarded as such, is now definitely music to the ears of my family, in particular my husband.

Another struggle that I initially had, was negotiating the staircase—after barely managing the first set of 6-7 steps, I had to stop and take a few good deep breaths before even contemplating completing the remaining steps. Finding a suitable position at nights to reduce the effects of the shortness of breath was nearly impossible during the initial period. I had to sleep in an upright position using about 5 pillows. I pondered the little luxury of being able to get into bed and lie in any position—this was impossible at that time! The physiological explanation is that the congestion of fluid in my lungs coupled with the limited amount of oxygen in the reduced amount of blood that my heart was managing to pump to my tissues resulted in significant shortness of breath and the fatigue I experienced. However, the problem with breathlessness has significantly improved with time and soon after, I was able to sleep in a more horizontal position with fewer pillows and not having the sensation of being drowned.

I was also feeling very lethargic—tired and washed out—even after the breathing difficulties had subsided. However, I have been able to gradually increase the amount of physical activities that I am able to do daily and I'm now back to using my 'maxi-climber' and doing a good deal of walking in my garden and nearby fields and parks.

I started doing very light housework, e.g. washing up few dishes and gradually built up to operating and removing clothes from the washing machine and dryer, to very light vacuuming (using a very light cordless vacuum cleaner).

Fortunately, I was not required to do any additional housework and my children are teenagers which removed the pressure of looking after younger children. However, if those are activities that need to be dealt with, you will need to get as much help as possible from family and friends and adhere to the advice from your cardiac rehabilitation or HF team and GP/other healthcare professionals involved in your care.

People worry about having sexual intercourse after an MI. I can't honestly say that this was one of my chief worries personally, but I have a husband who was not shy about voicing his worries regarding this area . . . in a sensitive manner, I hasten to add! This is an issue that may not be brought up but may worry individuals and their partners alike. Sex is like any other physical activity which will temporarily put a strain on the heart causing a rise in heart rate and blood pressure. The increased work of the heart may cause chest pain or breathlessness as with similar activities. However, this usually settles without any further problems and is deemed as safe as any other similar physical activity. As is the case with other physical activities, sexual activities should be undertaken incrementally as is suitable to the individual who has had an MI.

Other sex related problems that may be encountered includes loss of libido in either party, due to the stress of the MI and/or worry associated with it. These problems may also arise as a result of side effects from some of the new drugs including beta blockers which may cause erectile dysfunction (ED) especially in males or as a result of circulatory problems associated with the cardiovascular disease or newly diagnosed or existing diabetes. If you experience any of these difficulties after an MI, then you are strongly advised to seek help from your GP or from a nurse or doctor in your cardiac team.

Driving is an area where life-changing actions may be evident. Driving is usually restricted for a period after an MI. Each individual circumstance will dictate the terms and conditions for him/her and whether the DVLA will need to be informed. If one has adequate support and/or does not feel well enough to drive, then this may not be an issue. However, some people may be very reliant on driving in their day-day activities and may feel well enough to continue doing so, making it a challenge to adhere to the advice to initially avoid driving. I was advised not to drive for 4 weeks post MI. This was just about enough for me. It is advised that one's motor insurance company is informed about any heart condition and treatment he/she may have received as a result. Otherwise, the insurance may not be valid. My motor insurance company did not appear too bothered when we volunteered this information. However, my own feeling is that it is in our best interest to inform them anyway.

Closely aligned with driving is the consideration regarding returning to work. A sick note is usually required for one's employer/insurance company to cover the period during which you are off work. This is usually arranged by the hospital and/or your GP. Many people return to work about 4-6 weeks after an MI. However, some people may require a shorter or longer period depending on how well they are and the nature of their job. Some people may decide to change their job or even take early retirement, depending on their individual circumstances. I returned to work after 6 weeks but on a significantly reduced number of hours and doing much lighter duties. For me, this was beneficial, not just from a financial position but helped to improve my mental state and ongoing physical recovery. The key, though, is to be attuned to your body and 'listen' and respond appropriately to any alarms that may be sounding even at a low/subtle level.

Another of the activities that is affected following an MI is that of travelling by air and going on holidays, especially abroad. The decision about going on holiday is dependent on how you are physically as well as down to your preferences. Some people may prefer to wait until after they are fully recovered whilst others may find that being away from everything in a new/different environment on holidays augments their recovery process. It is usually safe to travel by air a few weeks after an uncomplicated MI. However, it is advised to wait until you feel fully recovered to travel by air and liaise with your GP and/or other members of the cardiac team. It is recommended that you check with the airline about the need to inform them about your heart condition. In addition, there will be implications for travelling with medications. You should pack an adequate supply and ensure any special rules governing any of your medications are adhered to. It is also recommended to travel with an up-to-date list of all the medications that you are being treated with in case any loss of medications or any other complications /problems occur. It is equally good practice to have a written summary of your medical history including the correct details of your cardiac problems and any intervention or surgery that was undertaken. The summary should also include any known drug allergies one may have. My own suggestion is a copy of your most recent hospital discharge summary and cardiac outpatient clinic letter. These usually contain all the above pertinent information. Needless to say, it is paramount that you have good/adequate travel insurance that will cover for any eventualities including complications from the heart problem. This inevitably, means increased costs but is worth arranging this properly prior to travelling. The BHF has a list of insurers deemed reputable for use by those of us in this situation. After all the above is arranged, it is very important, that we arrive at the airport in plenty of time to avoid rushing and unnecessary stress as well as allowing for any unforeseen eventualities!

My family planned a Caribbean holiday prior to my MI. The challenge is to see how things will work on a practical level when we do travel as planned. That will be a new experience for us all, but I am anticipating a smooth process as much as is possible by being well prepared including taking all necessary precautions.

Moving forward for a child of God means embracing my Christian teachings and principles. This requires faith in the teachings of the Bible, especially as a doctor who is aware of and understands the implications of the medical report.

In the Bible story in Numbers 13:30-33, the spies were challenged by Caleb about whose report they would believe. It was a decision to become terrified and paralysed by the report of the giant inhabitants of the Promised Land, though true and real, or taking the attitude that they had what it took, with God's support to defeat the giants—a task that seemed impossible to most. Only Caleb and Joshua, the two spies that subscribed to the latter position, were instrumental in the defeat and conquest of the 'Promised Land.' Biblical history tells us that they were the only two survivors of their generation that entered and inhabited Canaan along with their descendants. Similarly, I am determined to defeat those giants that this condition inevitably brings about. Though they are real, I choose to take the attitude that with God's help, along with all the medical provisions available and the relevant lifestyle changes/practices; I too will conquer these giants!

Jesus' disciples in Luke 5:5-6 also took the attitude that although the instruction He gave them did not seem plausible, especially, as it specifically contravened the rules and practices of their occupation, they would obey, stating "... nevertheless, at thy word ..." Consequently, they found themselves with results that exceeded their expectations!

Having adhered to the above, I expect to attain a truly good report—much better than my current medical report, realising Proverbs 15: 30 (KJV) "... a good report maketh the bones fat (healthy)". This will also reinforce God's counsel to us in Proverbs 3:5, to trust in the Lord with all our HEART; and lean not unto our own understanding.

CHAPTER 11

Fearfully And
Wonderfully Made

As a Christian medical practitioner (doctor), I recognise the complex nature of human beings as comprising a body, soul, and spirit. I am in awe of the wonderful bodies that each of us has been gifted and recognise the ongoing quest to unearth its intricate and amazing compilation and functioning.

In Psalm 139:14 (KJV), David, the psalmist wrote: "I am fearfully and wonderfully made, marvellous are thy works and that my soul knoweth right well". The concept of being fearfully and wonderfully made is for me a reassertion that I am purposefully designed and created and have been endowed with marvellous and astounding capacity. Inherent in this is the fact that I have been intelligently designed with order and form which clearly did not occur as a random event. My extensive studies of the human body have left me convinced that human beings are definitely not the product of chance or haphazard construction!

Many scientists attest to the wonder and order of the human creation, e.g. German-American rocket scientist and aerospace engineer, Wernher van Braun (1912–1977) stated, "Certainly there are those who argue that the universe evolved out of a random process, but what random process could produce marvels such as the brain of a man or the system of the human eye?" I would also add "... or indeed, the human heart and circulatory system?" American author and biochemist, Isaac Asimov (1919–1992), further stated that the human brain is "... the most complex and orderly arrangement of matter in the universe."

Blaise Pascal the renowned French Mathematician, Physicist and Catholic Theologian, after whom the pascal (Pa) SI unit of pressure is named (so says my engineer husband), gave an excellent description of the heart at a non-physical level. Pascal stated: "There is a God-shaped vacuum in the heart of every man which cannot be filled by any created thing, but only by God, the Creator, made known through Jesus."

Please do let me know, via www.fearfullyandwonderfully. org if you come across or know of other quotes regarding the heart from famous scientists that I may include on the website.

Such an appreciation of who one is and how one is made directly challenges the notion that we are merely accidental products of 'roll of the dice' evolutionary processes; hence the reason the theory of evolution is recognised as just that—a 'THEORY', unlike a LAW, such as Newton's Law of gravity, which has been proven scientifically.

A message such as the one promoted by the evolution theory erases the concept of us being fearfully and wonderfully made. It also attempts to erode one's feeling of being purposefully and deliberately created, predicating the use of words such as "average" or "okay" to describe oneself and a deep-seated belief that you are nothing special.

Many factors influence the way/s we view ourselves. These include the way we were nurtured and taught as well as our life experiences. When I was growing up in my remote, little district (village) in Jamaica, I was convinced that I was the prettiest girl in the village! Now, looking back I laugh aloud and wonder what on God's earth made me hold onto and believe that thought? It may be because I was a well behaved, polite Christian child with good academic aptitude. These were qualities of inner beauty that people in my community recognised, and valued, hence I was treated with love and respect and was well accepted.

Perhaps, I equated being loved, respected and accepted by my community with being pretty! After all, isn't this how society expects beautiful people to be treated? Beauty is by all accounts a universally accepted attribute. Whatever, the reason, such a feeling gave me a certain amount of self-confidence (even if I was unaware of the workings at the time), which has enabled me to believe in myself throughout life and has undoubtedly, impacted the person I am today. As a person who accepted and embraced the Christian faith from my early years, I was never left in any doubt that I am a unique and one of a kind individual.

Furthermore, my humble beginnings were never going to represent any barriers to me realising my potential. As far as I am concerned, my potential was already wrapped up in my DNA waiting to be realised!

Dr. Francis Collins, former head of The Human Genome Project and president of the US National Institute of Health, who is a renowned Christian scientist, describes the human genome as an individual's complete set of DNA containing all his/her genes. This may be described as an instruction book which is passed on from parent to child on how to build one unique human being ... like me ... or you! Thus, our genome is our unique recipe or our blueprint! This explains why DNA contains all the information that produces our phenotypical characteristics, such as our hair and eye colour and our height as well as our characteristic traits, our health and predisposition to illnesses.

The human genome project has revealed through DNA sequencing that the human genome is made up of around 3 billion letter combinations. There are four letters in the DNA alphabet, named after the four nucleotide bases of a DNA molecule—ACGT (Adenine, Cytosine, Guanine and Thymine). Hence, an individual's, genome is a sequence of A, C, G & T's in different sequences/patterns. This is equivalent to a stack of books about 61 metres high, made up of 200 books, each containing 500 pages with the letters A, C, G and T inscribed in various patterns and sequences! Reciting the contents of all 200 books in the stack would take around a century, if we recited one letter per second for 24 hours a day continually! If we were to extend our genome it would stretch about 3,000 kilometres (1,864 miles), or the distance from London to the Canary Islands!

What is even more amazing is the fact that the double-helix DNA strand is folded into the nucleus of each of the 37 trillion (37 million, million) cells in our body. To put this in perspective, if every cell in your body represents 1 second in time, then all your cells would represent 1.17 million years! Therefore, counting every cell in your body, multiplied by the number of letter combinations contained in the genome in each one of your cells, equates to 3,519 trillion years or 351.9 terabytes of data (this is around 700 laptops with 500GB hard drives)! Is this not proof that you are fearfully and wonderfully made?

Each cell contains the same genetic information; however, each cell uses this same information in a different way, e.g. a skin cell uses the information different to a cardiomyocyte (heart muscle cell). This points to the amazing and wonderful work of our creator. As a result of this fact, scientific development can make use of stem cell technology. Who knows, this may one day be applicable to the precision management of cardiac disease including post MI management, perhaps as it relates to the regeneration of cardiomyocytes! As discussed earlier in this book, there is ongoing research in this area.

No human being has a perfect genome. As Christians, we believe that God intended us all to be perfect but things went awry after the fall of man which brought on the Curse found in the Adam and Eve story in Genesis chapter 3. Yet, despite the defects from the various genetic errors, we function immensely well! Our 'instruction book' (DNA) contains 'typos' which may represent missing or corrupted information such as missing letters or sentences or duplications.

"For exmple this setence includes mising leters, mut8t1ons 4nd duuplications, but stilll makes sensse".

Although some of these 'typos' are common and benign, in other instances, a seemingly insignificant 'typo' may be responsible for serious pathological conditions, e.g. in two well-known conditions—Sickle Cell Anaemia and Cystic Fibrosis.

Sickle cell anaemia which occurs mostly in people of African or Mediterranean descent occurs as a result of a mutation in the beta haemoglobin gene. In this mutation, one amino acid is replaced by another in the beta globin chain causing an abnormally sickle-shaped red blood cell (when deoxygenated) and significant disruption in the normal functioning of the oxygen carrying molecule (haemoglobin) in our blood. The result is excessive destruction of these cells causing anaemia as well as occlusions (blockages) in blood vessels, joints and tissues from the abnormally shaped cells resulting in widespread ischaemia (lack-of blood supply) and tremendous suffering, simply because one protein (based on a sequence of DNA letter combinations) is out of place in the gene.

Cystic Fibrosis (CF) is also an example of a mutation that causes significant and far reaching problems to individuals with this problem, occurring predominantly in the Caucasian population. In CF, there is a mutation in the gene that makes a protein called Cystic Fibrosis Transmembrane (CFTR) causing abnormal or no CFTR protein. This causes the body to have thick, sticky mucus instead of the thin watery kind that we are accustomed to. This causes build-up of very thick mucus in various organs resulting in recurrent infections, particularly chest infections, digestive and fertility problems.

It is worth noting that cancers are also caused by mutations of the DNA.

I now wonder whether I possess a deletion or duplication or mutation in my DNA that renders my coronary blood vessels more susceptible to injury, resulting in me having had an MI when least expected. Of course, this is just a postulation but one worth exploring if deemed well-founded!

99.5% of the DNA of all human beings is similar and we are at most only 0.5% different from each other. However, this 0.5% difference in our DNA is responsible for us being unique individuals! My unique genome is what took me from the state of a single fertilised egg to the human being I am today! My parents came together, and each provided a gamete (sex cell, containing 23 chromosomes) to form me. The composition of the two gametes formed a zygote—a single fertilized cell which became a newly conceived human life. From that one cell within my mother's uterus developed all the various types of tissues, organs, and systems, all working together at just the right time in an amazingly coordinated and synchronised process to form a complete fully functional human being—me! Make no mistake; the journey that the gametes had to overcome to become me was no ordinary feat. Nonetheless, God ordained it that the two cells overcame all possible obstacles and came together to form Carol! All my systems came together by week 6-8 as a foetus.

Essentially, the human body is the most complex and unique organism. That complexity and uniqueness speaks volumes about the mind of its Creator. Every aspect of the body, down to the tiniest microscopic cell, reveals that it is fearfully and wonderfully made! Even the microscopic appearance of our DNA is a work of art! Dr Francis Collins, in one of his talks compared two slides at the end of one of his lectures. The similarity between the form, beauty, splendour and intricate details of each art work captivated the audience. He later revealed the first slide to be a photograph of the Rose window at the York Minster Cathedral in the UK; the second slide which shared a striking similarity to the first, was a cross section of the double helix DNA structure! Both amazing works of art!! (Links to illustrations of these artworks can be found from the accompanying website www.fearfullyandwonderfully.org).

If you consider yourself unremarkable or ordinary, you're not seeing yourself as God's divine creation. When we discover the truth that we are God's unique design, it is overwhelming. The truth is, "God created us in his own image (Genesis 1:27)".

God has fearfully and wonderfully made us, setting us apart as the brightest, clearest mirror of His creativity. While evolutionary biology considers us nothing more than glorified apes, scientific research confirms that humans are vastly unique on many levels e.g. only humans possess the ability to create and understand art and drawing[3].

Our capacity for abstract thinking sets us apart from animals. By referring to unobservable events and changes, we are

---

3 Klein, R.G. 1992. Evolutionary Anthropology 1: 5-14. and Balter, M. 1999. "Restorers reveal 28,000-year-old artworks". Science 283: 1835

able to formulate explanations of why certain things are happening. Chimpanzees, for example, operate in a world of concrete, tangible things merely reacting to conditioning from directly observable events[4].

In addition, humans are set apart from all other creatures by the ability to make moral judgments. We can discern between what is right and wrong. No animal models exist for human pride, shame, or guilt[5].

The fact that we have been provided with a manual (The Bible) is another testament to the deliberateness of our creator. We ignore that manual at our peril! Even though each of us has our unique blueprint; the mould broken and destroyed once we were made, the same manual applies to us all!

As human beings we are created to be kept healthy in our entirety, that is, in our trichotomous state. God cares about our total health! The Apostle John penned this wish in 1John1:3 (NKJV), stating "Beloved, I pray that you may prosper in all things and be in health, just as your soul prospers". Caring for our bodies is a spiritual discipline and an act of worship to God, as described in Romans 12:1 (KJV), by Apostle Paul who encourages each of us to present our bodies as "a living sacrifice, holy, acceptable unto God, which is your reasonable service".

---

4   Povinelli, D.J. 1998. "Animal Self-Awareness: A Debate Can Animals Empathize?" Scientific American

5   New Scientist 158(2134):19, May 16, 1998

So, next time you look in the mirror, see what God sees—
His marvellous creation! Fearfully and wonderfully made! A
fascinating design and masterpiece, of body, soul and spirit!
Appreciate who you are and recognise the urgency and
importance of looking after your physical body, including
your precious heart and your immortal soul and spirit. Let
your spirit nurture a true relationship with God and others
around you. Gaze in the mirror and say—"I am fearfully
and wonderfully made! Unique! One of a kind! Purposefully
and masterfully crafted! Designed to overcome life's biggest
challenges—even a heart attack!"

Friends and brethren listen up: "MY DREAM WAS
DISRUPTED . . . BUT IT DIDN'T DIE!" "My future
grandchildren, it's gonna be Jamaica here we come for those
amazing holidays, and wi travelling First Class style all de
way, Man!"

Glossary Of Terms

Abbrev.	Medical Term
A&E	Accident & Emergency
ACS	Acute Coronary Syndrome
ANS	Autonomic Nervous System
AV	Atrio-Ventricular
BCS	British Cardiovascular Society
BHF	British Heart Foundation
BMI	Body Mass Index
CABG	Coronary Artery Bypass Graft
CF	Cystic Fibrosis
CFTR	Cystic Fibrosis Transmembrane
CHD	Coronary Heart (Artery) Disease (Ischaemic Heart Disease)
CNS	Central Nervous System
CO	Cardiac Output
CPR	Cardiopulmonary Resuscitation
CVS	Cardiovascular System
DNA	Deoxyribonucleic Acid
DOH	Department of Health

Abbrev.	Medical Term
ECG	Electrocardiogram
ECHO	Echocardiogram
ED	Erectile Dysfunction
ENT	Ear, Nose and Throat
ESV	English Standard Version
FH	Familial Hypercholesterolaemia
GTN	Glycerine Trinitrate
HF	Heart Failure
HOCM	Hypertrophic Cardiomyopathy
ICD	Implantable Cardioverter Defibrillator
ISV	International Standard Version
IV	Intravenous
KJV	King James Version
LAD	Left Anterior Descending artery
LMCA	Left Main Coronary Artery
LQTS	Long QT Syndrome
LRI	Leicester Royal Infirmary
LVSD	Left Ventricular Systolic Dysfunction
MI	Myocardial Infarction (Heart Attack)
MINAP	The Myocardial Ischaemia National Audit Project
NET	New English Translation
NHS	National Health Service
NICE	The National Institute for Health and Care Excellence

Abbrev.	Medical Term
NIV	New International Version
NKJV	New King James Version
NSTEMI	None S T Elevation Myocardial Infarction
Pa	pascal—SI derived unit of pressure
PCCD	Progressive Cardiac Conduction Defect
PCI	Percutaneous Coronary Intervention
RCA	Right coronary artery
SA	Sino-Atrial
SADS	Sudden Arrhythmic Death Syndrome
S-ICD	Subcutaneous Implantable Cardioverter Defibrillator
STEMI	S T Elevation Myocardial Infarction
T2DM	Type 2 Diabetes Mellitus
VSD	Ventricular Septal Defect
WHO	World Health Organisation

About The Author

Carol is a General Medical Practitioner (GP/family doctor) in the United Kingdom. She was born in Jamaica where she grew up. Carol is married to Simon and they have two wonderful teenage sons.

Carol currently works as a sessional GP with leadership roles including 'Clinical Lead' & 'Clinical Supervisor'. Since qualifying as a GP, she has worked in primary care settings including GP surgeries; Urgent Care Centres; Out of Hours GP clinics and in a major Clinical Navigation Hub.

Carol's clinical experience in secondary care includes acute medicine, Diabetes care; care of the elderly, gastroenterology, stroke, psychiatry, paediatrics, obstetrics and gynaecology. She has also worked in medical research with a focus on Asthma, Diabetes and Cardiovascular Disease.

Her clinical repertoire also includes over 13 years of international nursing/midwifery experience prior to commencing training as a doctor. This included the role of Practice Nurse with responsibility for managing chronic illnesses including Coronary Heart Disease.

Carol enjoys Public Speaking and giving presentations. She has won two awards for 'Best Speaker' in National Nurses' Week events and has had the opportunity to present research and clinical audit findings at International Medical Conferences. She also volunteers her time to deliver presentations on various health matters to small and large groups at local, regional and national church and community events.

In the non-clinical setting, Carol volunteers as Secretary for a local charity, serves as President for her church's Women's Ministry Department, as an Adult Sunday School Teacher and a member of the church's Praise and Worship Team. She still hopes to resume her piano lessons to become a 'decent' player. Carol is passionate about her friends and family with whom she likes to enjoy a 'good belly laugh'.

The aforementioned roles and experiences have equipped Carol with a wide range of clinical and social skills and competencies. These attributes, along with her recent health related 'escapade', qualify Carol as an authority on how a heart attack impacts holistic health.

Printed in Great Britain
by Amazon

33925765R00070